Sara Wells

Arcturian Healing Methods
A Journey Through Multidimensional
Healing

Original Title: Métodos de Cura Arcturiana

Copyright © 2024, published by Luiz Antonio dos Santos ME.

This book is a work of non-fiction that explores practices and concepts in the field of multidimensional and energy healing. Through a comprehensive approach, the author offers practical tools to understand Arcturian principles, promote energy balance, and access higher frequencies of healing and transformation.

1st Edition

Production Team:
Author: Sara Wells
Editor: Luiz Santos
Revision: Gloria Santos
Cover: Studios Booklas / Serge Mills
Layout: Armando Telles
Translation: Gustavo Soler
Publication and Identification

Arcturian Healing Methods
Booklas, 2025
Categories: Psychology / Spirituality / Energy Healing
DDC: 158.1 - CDU: 615.851
All rights reserved to:
Luiz Antonio dos Santos ME / Booklas

No part of this book may be reproduced, stored in a retrieval system, or transmitted by any means—electronic, mechanical, photocopy, 1 recording, or otherwise—without 2 the prior and express permission of the copyright holder.

Summary

Prologue 6
Chapter 1 Arcturians and Healing... 8
Chapter 2 Energy Anatomy.. 12
Chapter 3 Preparation for Healing 16
Chapter 4 Multidimensional Healing.. 21
Chapter 5 Energy Surgery.. 26
Chapter 6 Arcturian Crystals.. 31
Chapter 7 Arcturian Symbols... 35
Chapter 8 Arcturian Meditation 38
Chapter 9 Conscious Breathing.. 42
Chapter 10 Healing Sounds.. 46
Chapter 11 Arcturian Chromotherapy.. 50
Chapter 12 DNA Activation 54
Chapter 13 Healing the Past... 58
Chapter 14 Healing the Present.. 62
Chapter 15 Healing the Future 66
Chapter 16 Healing the Physical Body 70
Chapter 17 Emotional Healing... 74
Chapter 18 Mental Healing.. 78
Chapter 19 Spiritual Healing.. 81
Chapter 20 Soul Healing.. 85
Chapter 21 Healing the Planet 88
Chapter 22 Distance Healing 92
Chapter 23 Arcturian Technology.. 96

- Chapter 24 Quantum Leap 100
- Chapter 25 Astral Travel 104
- Chapter 26 Arcturian Communication 108
- Chapter 27 Healing with Masters 112
- Chapter 28 Healing with Angels 116
- Chapter 29 Healing with Animals 120
- Chapter 30 Healing with Plants 124
- Chapter 31 Healing for Children 128
- Chapter 32 Healing for Couples 132
- Chapter 33 Healing for Family 135
- Chapter 34 Healing for Animals 139
- Chapter 35 Healing for the Environment 143
- Chapter 36 Healing for Businesses 146
- Chapter 37 Planetary Healing and Ascension 150
- Chapter 38 Awakening of Consciousness 154
- Chapter 39 Soul Purpose 157
- Chapter 40 Intuition and Inner Guidance 161
- Chapter 41 Self-Healing and Self-Knowledge 165
- Chapter 42 Forgiveness and Compassion 169
- Chapter 43 Gratitude and Abundance 173
- Chapter 44 Manifestation and Co-creation 176
- Chapter 45 Energy Exercises 180
- Chapter 46 Mantras and Affirmations 184
- Chapter 47 Creative Visualizations 188
- Chapter 48 Arcturian Rituals 192
- Chapter 49 Arcturian Cards 196
- Chapter 50 Ethics in Healing 200

Chapter 51 Healing and the Ascension Process 204
Chapter 52 Arcturian Community 208
Chapter 53 Next Steps in Arcturian Healing 212
Chapter 54 Arcturian Masters 216
Chapter 55 The Future of Healing 220

Prologue

You are about to enter a universe that resonates beyond logic and the tangible. The words that follow in this book are not just information, but vibrational keys to awaken something deep within you—something that already exists, but remains dormant. This book, with its pages imbued with subtle energies, did not come to you by chance. There is a hidden purpose in your choice to hold it now, perhaps a call from your own higher self, which recognizes the truth in each word even before they are read.

Within these pages lies an ancient technology, a knowledge that transcends ages and dimensions. Here, the Arcturians, masters of multidimensional healing, share their tools for you to access a level of balance and harmony rarely found in earthly experience. Each method, each technique described is not just a healing practice, but an invitation for you to align yourself with the highest frequencies of love, light, and expansion.

The Arcturians, beings of unparalleled wisdom, are not separate from you; they are reflections of your own divine essence. The healing they offer is not something external, but a catalyst for you to awaken the healer within yourself. In the following pages, you will find not only methods, but portals—tools to access dimensions where the impossible dissolves and true healing occurs. Imagine yourself flowing between the layers of your own being, clearing blockages, healing old wounds, awakening dormant potentials, and experiencing a transformation that reverberates on all levels of your existence.

What is here is for you, exclusively for you, because what needs to be awakened is unique and personal. Each line you read will activate something different on your journey. This book is not a manual; it is an experience, a reconnection with the universal energy that sustains everything. The practices described here transcend the limits of the rational mind and connect you with a cosmic intelligence that already knows what you need.

Allow yourself to dive in. Open yourself to receive. The Arcturian knowledge you are about to access has the power to transform not only your life, but the world around you. Because when you raise your frequency, you become a light that illuminates everything you touch. This is the call that brought you here. This is the time to respond.

Sincerely: Luiz Santos
Editor

Chapter 1
Arcturians and Healing

The universe of Arcturian healing is revealed as a dimension of extraordinary possibilities, leading to a transformative experience that transcends the limitations of earthly existence. Based on high principles of unconditional love, energy balance, and expansion of consciousness, this practice connects us to a civilization of highly evolved beings, the Arcturians. Inhabitants of a higher vibrational frequency, they use their ancient wisdom to assist humanity in the ascension process, promoting the harmonization of the physical, emotional, mental, and spiritual bodies. This interaction is not just an exchange of knowledge, but a journey of integration and reconnection with the divine essence that resides in each human being.

The Arcturians are described as beings of light, whose physical appearance symbolizes their direct connection to the cosmos: tall, with blue skin and deep eyes that reflect their infinite wisdom. However, it is their energetic and telepathic presence that impacts the most, allowing them to communicate directly with the subtle fields of individuals. In their healing practices, they use advanced technologies that work with the manipulation of frequencies and energy, restoring the natural balance of being and eliminating blockages that compromise the vital flow. These processes not only alleviate physical symptoms but also promote an internal transformation, allowing access to higher dimensions of consciousness.

The essence of Arcturian healing is rooted in a deep understanding of the multidimensionality of the human being. By recognizing that diseases and imbalances originate in the energy bodies before manifesting physically, the Arcturians teach us the importance of looking beyond the visible. Through techniques that raise vibration and reprogram limiting patterns, they create a solid foundation for integral healing. In this process, unconditional love emerges as a central element, not only as a catalyst for transformation but also as an invitation for each to discover their own inner light and empower their evolutionary path.

This practice is more than a healing approach; it is a philosophy of life that expands the perception of reality and awakens a deep sense of purpose. By working in harmony with the Arcturians, individuals experience not only the release of traumas and negative beliefs but also the reconnection with their highest essence. This movement generates benefits ranging from physical and emotional healing to spiritual growth, promoting a full integration between mind, body, and spirit. It is a call for humanity to align with the highest frequencies of light and love, thus traversing the path of its true evolution.

Inhabitants of the star Arcturus, in the constellation Boötes, the Arcturians are an evolved civilization that vibrates in a dimension higher than ours. Their history goes back millions of years, and their wisdom has accumulated through countless ages of learning and spiritual evolution. They are beings of pure light and unconditional love, dedicated to assisting humanity on its path of ascension.

The Arcturians present themselves as tall and slender beings, with bluish skin and large almond-shaped eyes that emanate deep wisdom. Their communication transcends verbal language, transmitting messages telepathically, through images, feelings, and ideas. They master advanced technologies that use energy and vibration for healing, transportation, and interdimensional communication. Their starships, true works of art of cosmic engineering, are capable of traversing dimensional portals and manipulating space-time.

Arcturian healing philosophy is based on the principle that we are multidimensional beings, composed of body, mind, and spirit, and that disease manifests first in the subtle bodies before materializing in the physical body. Through the manipulation of energy, the Arcturians act on the subtle energy fields, removing blockages, repairing traumas, and restoring the natural balance of being.

Arcturian healing is intrinsically linked to spiritual ascension, a process of raising consciousness that leads us to union with the Divine. By balancing our energy bodies and releasing limiting patterns, Arcturian healing propels us on this evolutionary journey, awakening our latent potential and expanding our consciousness.

Basic principles of Arcturian healing:

Energy: Arcturian healing recognizes energy as the foundation of all life and uses techniques to manipulate and direct this energy to promote healing and well-being.

Vibration: Each being and object has a unique vibrational frequency. Arcturian healing seeks to raise the vibration of the individual, harmonizing it with higher frequencies of love and light.

Consciousness: Arcturian healing emphasizes the importance of consciousness in the healing process. By becoming aware of our limiting patterns and negative beliefs, we can transform them and create a healthier and happier reality.

Multidimensionality: Arcturian healing works on all levels of being: physical, emotional, mental, and spiritual. This holistic approach aims at the integral healing of the individual.

Unconditional Love: Unconditional love is the foundation of Arcturian healing. The Arcturians emanate unconditional love in all their actions, creating an environment of healing and compassion.

Benefits of Arcturian healing:

Physical Healing: Relieves pain, accelerates recovery from illness, strengthens the immune system, and promotes rejuvenation.

Emotional Healing: Releases traumas, fears, anxiety, depression, and other emotional imbalances, promoting inner peace and emotional well-being.

Mental Healing: Increases mental clarity, focus, concentration, and creativity. It helps in overcoming negative thought patterns and limiting beliefs.

Spiritual Healing: Awakens consciousness, strengthens the connection with the Higher Self, accelerates the ascension process, and promotes spiritual growth.

Expansion of Consciousness: Expands the perception of reality, increases intuition, and opens the way for the development of psychic abilities.

Harmony and Balance: Promotes energy balance on all levels, restoring harmony between body, mind, and spirit.

Self-knowledge: Facilitates the process of self-knowledge, helping in the identification of limiting patterns and in the development of inner potential.

Connection with the Arcturians: Strengthens the connection with the Arcturians and their teachings, opening the way for guidance and assistance on your evolutionary journey.

Thus, Arcturian healing is revealed as a profound path of transformation and reconnection, where the harmonization between body, mind, and spirit leads to the awakening of our true essence. This practice transcends techniques, offering an experience of elevation and expansion, guided by the wisdom of beings dedicated to assisting humanity on its evolutionary journey.

Chapter 2
Energy Anatomy

The human energy anatomy is a complex and interconnected system that sustains our existence on multiple levels, providing the foundation for health, well-being, and spiritual evolution. Composed of subtle bodies, chakras, and meridians, this structure is not just a reflection of the physical body, but the matrix that directly influences our emotional, mental, and spiritual experiences. Understanding this anatomy is fundamental to accessing healing methods, such as the Arcturian approach, which works precisely with these energy fields to promote balance and integral harmonization.

The subtle bodies, which go beyond the physical plane, constitute different dimensions of our existence. The etheric body, closest to the physical, is responsible for sustaining vitality and forming an energy template that reflects and influences the state of health. The emotional body, on the other hand, holds our emotions and feeling patterns, being the key to understanding the origins of emotional blockages. The mental body, in turn, organizes thoughts and beliefs that shape the perception of reality, while the spiritual body connects us to the divine and the highest essence, enabling intuitive insights and the expansion of consciousness. Each of these energy layers plays an essential role in the overall harmony of the being.

The chakras, energy centers located along the body, function as portals for transformation and distribution of vital energy. Each of the seven main chakras is associated with specific aspects of our existence, from the most basic needs, such as security and survival, to the highest dimensions, such as spirituality and enlightenment. The balance of each chakra is essential for the healthy functioning of organs, glands and systems, in addition to directly reflecting our emotional and mental states. An unbalanced chakra can limit the flow of energy, affecting both physical health and personal development.

Furthermore, the energy meridians act as channels that connect different parts of the system, allowing vital energy to flow throughout the body. When there are blockages or interruptions in these pathways, symptoms arise ranging from fatigue and physical illness to emotional instability and spiritual disconnection. Restoring this energy flow is essential to regaining balance, and practices such as Arcturian healing act directly on removing blockages, using high frequencies and vibrations to re-establish harmony between body, mind and spirit.

This understanding of energy anatomy opens pathways to a new perception of health and well-being, inviting us to explore the deeper dimensions of being. By recognizing the interdependence between our energy layers and physical manifestations, we can address imbalances holistically, promoting a transformation that goes beyond physical healing and reaches the essence of our being.

Just as we have a physical body with organs, bones and tissues, we also have an energy body composed of different layers and subtle structures. These layers, known as subtle bodies, interact with each other and with the physical body, influencing our health and well-being in a profound way.

Subtle Bodies:
- **Etheric Body:** It is the layer closest to the physical body, a kind of "energy template" that supports the vitality and health of the physical body.
- **Emotional Body:** It houses our emotions, feelings and emotional patterns. Imbalances in this body can manifest as anxiety, fear, anger or sadness.
- **Mental Body:** It is the home of our thoughts, beliefs and mental patterns. Negative thoughts and limiting beliefs can generate energy blocks and affect our health.

- **Spiritual Body:** It connects us with our divine essence, our Higher Self and the spiritual plane. Through this body, we access intuition, inner wisdom and connection with the Divine.

Chakras:

Chakras are vortices of energy that capture, transform and distribute vital energy (prana) throughout the body. They are like "wheels" that spin at different speeds and directions, influencing the functioning of the organs, glands and systems of the physical body. There are seven main chakras located along the spine, each with a specific color, function and vibration:

1. **Root Chakra (Muladhara):** Located at the base of the spine, related to security, survival and connection to Earth.
2. **Sacral Chakra (Svadhisthana):** Located in the lower abdomen, related to creativity, sexuality, emotions and pleasure.
3. **Solar Plexus Chakra (Manipura):** Located in the stomach area, related to personal power, self-esteem, will and identity.
4. **Heart Chakra (Anahata):** Located in the center of the chest, related to love, compassion, forgiveness and connection with others.
5. **Throat Chakra (Vishuddha):** Located in the throat, related to communication, expression and creativity.
6. **Third Eye Chakra (Ajna):** Located between the eyebrows, related to intuition, wisdom, inner vision and perception.
7. **Crown Chakra (Sahasrara):** Located at the top of the head, related to spirituality, connection with the Divine and enlightenment.

Meridians:

Meridians are energy channels that run throughout the body, conducting vital energy and connecting organs and systems with each other. Acupuncture and other traditional Chinese medicine techniques work with the meridians to restore the flow of energy and promote healing.

Energy Imbalances:
When the flow of energy is blocked or unbalanced, physical, emotional and spiritual problems can arise. Traumas, negative emotions, limiting thoughts and challenging experiences can generate energy blocks that affect health and well-being. Arcturian healing works on these blockages, removing them and restoring the natural flow of vital energy.

How to identify energy imbalances:
- **Diseases and physical symptoms:** Pain, fatigue, insomnia, digestive problems, allergies and other health conditions can indicate energy imbalances.
- **Emotional imbalances:** Anxiety, depression, fear, anger, irritability and other negative emotional states can be signs of blockages in the emotional body.
- **Negative mental patterns:** Obsessive thoughts, limiting beliefs, difficulty concentrating and lack of mental clarity can indicate imbalances in the mental body.
- **Spiritual disconnection:** Feeling of existential emptiness, lack of purpose, difficulty connecting with the Divine and loss of faith can indicate blockages in the spiritual body.

Recognizing and working with energy anatomy is not just a tool for healing, but an invitation to a journey of self-discovery and profound transformation. As we delve into these subtle aspects of our existence, we are called to integrate body, mind and spirit in a harmonious movement that resonates with the highest purpose of our soul. It is in this alignment that we find not only health, but also full realization and connection with the whole, allowing our energy to flow freely as a reflection of universal balance.

Chapter 3
Preparation for Healing

Preparing for healing is an act of profound intention and alignment, where each element of body, mind and spirit is adjusted to receive the transforming frequencies that the Arcturians offer. This process begins with the creation of a sacred space that functions as an energy refuge. More than a physical place, this environment must vibrate in harmony with your intention to heal, promoting tranquility and receptivity. For this, it is essential to purify the space, both physically and energetically, using practices such as organizing the environment, using incense or crystals, and visualizing light energies filling the place. This initial preparation symbolizes the opening of a portal to a deeper connection with Arcturian energies.

Contact with the Arcturians requires a state of presence and gratitude. This connection is not limited to words or rituals, but involves the tuning of the heart with frequencies of love and compassion. An effective way to invoke them is by combining words with visualizations, imagining a luminous field that expands around you and connects to higher dimensions. This interaction is deeply strengthened when anchored in clear intentions, expressed through affirmations or mantras. Imagine a flow of energy descending from the cosmos, filling you with light as the Arcturians emanate wisdom and healing directly to your energy field. This moment of openness is also an opportunity to cultivate feelings of humility and respect, essential for interacting with these elevated beings.

Energy protection is another indispensable component in preparation. Visualizing firm roots connecting you to the Earth creates a sense of stability, while imagining a shield of light around the body establishes a barrier against unwanted external influences. These simple practices, combined with the invocation of spirit guides, not only ensure energy security, but also strengthen the feeling of being enveloped by a loving and protective energy. This shield of light, constantly renewed by your intention and connection with the Arcturians, is a powerful tool to maintain clarity and focus during the healing process.

Through the combination of conscious breathing, creative visualization and setting intentions, the individual tunes in more deeply with Arcturian energy. Breathing acts as a channel that harmonizes the physical body with the subtle bodies, while visualization directs the flow of energy to the areas that need attention. Imagine the healing energy entering your body like a golden light, flowing to every cell, dissolving blockages and restoring balance. Additionally, practices such as meditation, relaxing music, aromatherapy and the use of crystals can further amplify your receptivity, creating an environment of total alignment for healing.

This preparation process is not just an initial step, but a path that strengthens the bond with higher energies and creates a solid foundation for lasting results. By adopting these practices with consistency and dedication, you transform the act of healing yourself into a rich journey of self-knowledge and spiritual ascension, expanding your ability to integrate the high frequencies of Arcturian healing.

Creating a Sacred Space:

The first step to prepare for Arcturian healing is to create a sacred space, a sanctuary of peace and tranquility where you can connect with the healing energy. This space can be a room in your home, a special corner in your bedroom, or even a place in nature that brings you peace and serenity.

Purifying the Environment:

- **Physical cleaning:** Start by cleaning the physical space, removing any objects that cause distraction or

disharmony. Vacuum, dust and organize the environment to create an atmosphere of order and cleanliness.
- **Energy purification:** Use energy purification techniques to cleanse the space of dense and stagnant energies. You can use incense, smudging, herbal sprays, crystals or sound to purify the environment.
- **Setting Intention:** Set the intention to create a sacred space for healing and connection with the Arcturians. Visualize the space filled with light, love and healing energies.

Invoking the Arcturians:

After preparing the physical space, it is time to invoke the presence of the Arcturians and request their assistance in the healing process. Do this with reverence and gratitude, acknowledging their wisdom and unconditional love.
- **Heart connection:** Connect with your heart, the center of love and compassion, and emanate feelings of gratitude and receptivity to the Arcturians.
- **Verbalization:** Use words to invoke the Arcturians, expressing your desire to receive their healing and guidance. You can use a prayer, a mantra or simply say aloud or mentally: "Beloved Arcturians, I humbly ask for your presence and assistance in this time of healing."
- **Visualization:** Visualize a portal of light opening in your sacred space and the Arcturians coming into contact with you, surrounding you with their loving and healing energy.

Energy Protection:

Before starting any healing practice, it is essential to protect your energy field from negative influences and dense energies.
- **Grounding:** Imagine roots coming out of your feet and penetrating deep into the Earth, connecting you with the planet's vital energy and providing stability and security.

- **Shield of light:** Visualize a shield of white or golden light surrounding your entire body, protecting you from any negative energy or interference.
- **Invocation of protection:** Invoke the protection of the Arcturians, angels or spirit guides, asking them to help you keep your energy field protected during the healing practice.

Intention, Visualization and Breathing:

Intention, visualization and conscious breathing are powerful tools that amplify the power of Arcturian healing.

- **Clear intention:** Clearly define your intention for healing, be it physical, emotional, mental or spiritual. The clearer and more specific your intention, the more powerful the healing will be.
- **Creative visualization:** Use visualization to direct healing energy to specific areas of your body or to situations that need healing. Imagine Arcturian energy flowing through you, removing blockages and restoring balance.
- **Conscious breathing:** Breathing is the bridge between the physical body and the energy body. Breathe deeply and consciously, allowing the healing energy to penetrate every cell of your being.

Other preparation practices:

- **Meditation:** Meditation calms the mind, harmonizes emotions and raises vibration, creating a receptive state for Arcturian healing.
- **Relaxing music:** Listening to soft, harmonious music helps create a relaxing atmosphere conducive to healing.
- **Aromatherapy:** Using essential oils with calming and purifying properties can aid in preparation for healing.
- **Crystals:** Using crystals that amplify healing energy, such as rose quartz, amethyst and selenite, can enhance the effects of Arcturian healing.

Preparation for healing is, in essence, a practice of inner alignment that transcends the physical and energetic steps described. It is an act of surrender and trust in the process, a genuine openness to receive the energies of transformation and balance. By dedicating yourself to these preparations with intention and presence, you not only lay the foundation for healing, but also reaffirm your commitment to yourself and your spiritual journey. In this sacred space created within and without you, the connection with the Arcturians becomes a vibrant exchange of light and love, reflecting the power of alignment between the human and the divine.

Chapter 4
Multidimensional Healing

Multidimensional healing transcends the conventional limits of healing, reaching the various layers that constitute the human being. This process encompasses physical, emotional, mental, and spiritual dimensions, promoting a profound and comprehensive balance. Imagine each aspect of your being as part of an interconnected network: when you take care of a specific point, the impact reverberates throughout the entire structure, restoring harmony. Through the elevated energy of the Arcturians, masters in the manipulation of vibrational frequencies, it is possible to rebalance each of these dimensions, bringing relief and well-being on multiple levels. This holistic approach not only treats symptoms but also eliminates blockages at their energetic origin, promoting lasting transformation.

On the physical plane, multidimensional healing works on cell regeneration, elimination of toxins, and strengthening the immune system. However, its action is not restricted to the material body. On emotional levels, Arcturian energy releases traumas and negative patterns, restoring inner peace and allowing feelings of love and compassion to flow freely. In the mental field, limiting beliefs and self-sabotaging thoughts are dissolved, creating space for a state of clarity, positivity, and focus. On the spiritual level, this healing facilitates the connection with the Higher Self, promoting the awakening of your divine essence and aligning you with your life mission.

The application of this technique involves simple but profoundly effective practices that harmonize mind, body, and spirit. By connecting with Arcturian energy, a flow of healing light is directed to the areas in need, whether through the laying on of hands, creative visualization, or the use of crystals and symbols. This process is amplified by clear intention and attunement to the high frequencies of the Arcturians, who guide and enhance each stage of healing. Furthermore, continuous practice not only generates immediate benefits but also stimulates self-knowledge and spiritual evolution, allowing you to better understand your own patterns and challenges.

This multidimensional approach is more than a healing method: it is a journey of transformation and growth, which redefines the way you perceive your health and well-being. By integrating Arcturian energy into your life, you not only heal existing imbalances, but also strengthen your connection to universal consciousness, expanding your ability to live in harmony with yourself and the world around you. It is an invitation to expand your vision of healing and align with your highest potential.

Arcturian Multidimensional Healing is an advanced technique that works on the different levels of being, promoting balance and harmonization in all dimensions. Imagine a vibrant and interconnected fabric, where each thread represents a dimension of your existence. When one thread becomes unbalanced, the entire fabric is affected. Multidimensional Healing aims to restore harmony in this fabric, bringing balance and well-being to all areas of your life.

Levels of Action of Multidimensional Healing:
1. **Physical Healing:** On the physical level, Arcturian Multidimensional Healing acts directly on the cellular structure of the body, promoting tissue regeneration, strengthening the immune system, and releasing toxins. Diseases and physical imbalances are treated at their root, considering the underlying energetic causes.
2. **Emotional Healing:** On the emotional level, Multidimensional Healing focuses on releasing traumas, fears, anxiety, anger, and other limiting emotional patterns. Through Arcturian energy, blocked emotions are

released and healed, bringing relief, inner peace, and emotional balance.
3. **Mental Healing:** On the mental level, Multidimensional Healing works on reprogramming limiting beliefs, negative thought patterns, and mental conditioning that hinder your growth and development. The mind is freed from patterns of scarcity, fear, and self-sabotage, opening space for abundance, prosperity, and personal fulfillment.
4. **Spiritual Healing:** On the spiritual level, Multidimensional Healing promotes connection with the Higher Self, the awakening of consciousness, and the expansion of your divine essence. Blockages that hinder your spiritual growth are removed, allowing you to connect with your life mission and express your full potential.

How to Apply Multidimensional Healing:

The application of Arcturian Multidimensional Healing involves the combination of different techniques, such as the laying on of hands, visualization, the use of Arcturian crystals and symbols, energy channeling, and telepathic communication with the Arcturians.

Step-by-step for applying Multidimensional Healing:
1. **Preparation:** Prepare the environment and yourself following the steps described in the previous chapter (Chapter 3: Preparation for Healing).
2. **Intention:** Clearly define your intention for healing, specifying the levels (physical, emotional, mental, and/or spiritual) on which you wish to act.
3. **Invocation:** Invoke the presence of the Arcturians and request their assistance in applying Multidimensional Healing.
4. **Connection:** Connect with the Arcturian energy, visualizing a flow of loving and healing light surrounding you and the person who will receive the healing (if applicable).

5. **Techniques:** Use the techniques you feel most guided to apply, such as:
   - **Laying on of Hands:** Place your hands on the person (or on yourself) and visualize Arcturian energy flowing through your hands, directing it to the areas that need healing.

   Visualization: Visualize Arcturian energy acting on the different levels of being, removing blockages, healing wounds, and restoring balance.

   Crystals: Use Arcturian crystals to amplify healing energy and direct it to specific areas.

   Symbols: Draw or visualize Arcturian symbols to activate healing codes and raise vibration.

   Channeling: Channel Arcturian energy through your body, allowing it to flow freely and act where needed.

   Telepathic Communication: Communicate telepathically with the Arcturians, requesting guidance and assistance during the healing process.

6. **Gratitude:** Thank the Arcturians for their presence and assistance in healing.
7. **Integration:** After applying Multidimensional Healing, take some time to integrate the healing energy, relaxing and observing the sensations and changes that occur in your body and mind.

Benefits of Multidimensional Healing:

- **Deep and comprehensive healing:** Acts on all levels of being, promoting physical, emotional, mental, and spiritual healing.
- **Balance and harmonization:** Restores energy balance in all dimensions, bringing harmony to your life.
- **Release of blockages:** Removes energy blockages that hinder your growth and development.
- **Expansion of consciousness:** Raises your vibration and expands your consciousness, opening the way for spiritual awakening.

- **Connection with the Higher Self:** Strengthens the connection with your Higher Self and your divine essence.
- **Self-knowledge:** Facilitates the process of self-knowledge, helping in understanding your patterns and challenges.
- **Personal transformation:** Promotes personal transformation and growth in all areas of your life.

Arcturian Multidimensional Healing is a powerful tool for healing and transformation. By mastering this technique, you can help yourself and others achieve balance, health, and well-being on all levels of being. In the next chapters, we will explore other Arcturian healing techniques and learn how to apply them in different situations.

Chapter 5
Energy Surgery

Arcturian energy surgery is a revolutionary practice that transcends conventional healing methods, offering a profoundly transformative approach through the manipulation of energy frequencies. This process, conducted by the Arcturians, operates on the subtle bodies of the human being, identifying and removing energy blockages, repairing damage, and restoring the harmonious flow of vital energy. Without the need for physical instruments, scalpels, or medications, this technique works precisely and effectively, achieving levels of physical, emotional, mental, and spiritual healing that profoundly impact health and well-being.

The Arcturians utilize sophisticated and highly vibrational tools to perform this healing technique. Lights of specific frequencies, emanating different colors and intensities, are directed to dissolve stagnant energies and stimulate cell regeneration. High vibration sounds are applied to defragment imbalance patterns, while advanced etheric technologies, such as energy lasers and healing crystals, operate on the subtle energy fields, promoting detailed adjustments and deep alignments. Visualization, both by the Arcturians and the recipient of the healing, enhances the process by creating a field of focused intention that amplifies the results.

The process follows an orderly and meticulous structure. It begins with a detailed energy diagnosis, where the Arcturians identify the origin of the imbalances and determine the blockages to be treated. Next, the recipient is energetically anchored and protected, ensuring safety throughout the session. After removing the blockages and clearing the dense patterns, Arcturian energy acts to repair the subtle bodies and regenerate the energy tissues. The process ends with the harmonization of all energy layers and the integration of healing energy, ensuring that the effects are assimilated completely and lastingly.

The benefits of this technique are broad and comprehensive. By treating not only the symptoms but also the underlying causes of diseases, energy surgery promotes deeper and more effective healing. Furthermore, the non-invasive nature of the procedure ensures a pain-free experience and physical recovery, making it accessible and safe. This multidimensional approach not only balances the physical aspects of being but also strengthens the energy field, preventing future illnesses and promoting a state of balance and vitality. At the same time, by raising vibration and expanding consciousness, it assists in spiritual awakening, connecting the individual with their divine essence and full potential.

When preparing for this transformative experience, it is essential to cultivate a clear intention and establish a state of receptivity. Creating a conducive environment, relaxing, and opening yourself to Arcturian energy facilitates connection and maximizes results. During the procedure, physical and emotional sensations may vary, including heat, vibrations, or even deep insights, reflecting the intensity and scope of the healing being performed. This interaction is not only a therapeutic process but also an invitation to a deeper connection with universal wisdom and the unconditional love of the Arcturians, inaugurating a path of lasting transformation and balance.

Arcturian Energy Surgery is a non-invasive technique that uses energy to act directly on the subtle bodies, promoting healing on deep levels. The Arcturians, with their advanced technology and knowledge of energy anatomy, are able to identify and remove energy blockages, dissolve disease patterns, repair damage to subtle bodies, and restore the natural flow of vital energy.

Tools and Techniques:

The Arcturians utilize a variety of tools and techniques to perform Energy Surgery, including:

- **Light:** Light is one of the main tools used by the Arcturians. They project rays of light of different colors and frequencies to remove blockages, dissolve negative energies, and promote healing.
- **Sound:** Specific sound frequencies are used to harmonize the subtle bodies, undo disease patterns, and stimulate cell regeneration.
- **Arcturian Technology:** The Arcturians use advanced instruments and technologies, such as etheric lasers, healing crystals, and energy probes, to perform precise surgical procedures on subtle bodies.
- **Etheric Hands:** The Arcturians can use their etheric hands to manipulate energy, remove blockages, and perform repairs on the subtle bodies.
- **Visualization:** Visualization is a powerful tool used by both the Arcturians and the patient to direct healing energy and enhance the effects of surgery.

How Arcturian Energy Surgery Works:

1. **Diagnosis:** The Arcturians perform a precise energy diagnosis, identifying the root cause of the problem and the energy blockages that need to be removed.
2. **Anchoring and Protection:** The patient is anchored to the Earth and energetically protected to ensure their safety and stability during the process.
3. **Removal of Blockages:** The Arcturians use their tools and techniques to remove energy blockages, dissolve negative energies, and disease patterns.
4. **Repair and Regeneration:** Arcturian energy is used to repair damage to subtle bodies, regenerate tissues, and restore the natural flow of vital energy.
5. **Harmonization and Integration:** The subtle bodies are harmonized, and the healing energy is integrated into all levels of being.

Benefits of Arcturian Energy Surgery:
- **Deep and accelerated healing:** Arcturian Energy Surgery promotes healing on deep levels, accelerating the recovery and regeneration process.
- **Non-invasive treatment:** It is a non-invasive technique, with no cuts, pain, or need for post-surgical recovery.
- **Removal of the root cause:** It acts on the root cause of the problem, removing energy blockages and disease patterns.
- **Multidimensional healing:** Promotes healing on all levels of being: physical, emotional, mental, and spiritual.
- **Disease prevention:** By removing energy blockages and strengthening the energy field, Arcturian Energy Surgery prevents the onset of diseases.
- **Awakening of consciousness:** Increases vibration and expands consciousness, assisting in the process of spiritual awakening.

How to Prepare for Arcturian Energy Surgery:
- **Clear intention:** Clearly define your intention for healing and the results you want to achieve.
- **Trust and surrender:** Trust the wisdom and unconditional love of the Arcturians, surrendering to the healing process.
- **Preparing the environment:** Create a sacred space, free from distractions and dense energies.
- **Relaxation and receptivity:** Relax your body and mind, opening yourself to receive the healing energy of the Arcturians.
- **Visualization:** Visualize Arcturian energy acting on your body, removing blockages and promoting healing.

Arcturian Energy Surgery Experience:

During Arcturian Energy Surgery, you may experience different sensations, such as heat, tingling, vibrations, pressure, or lightness. You may also have visions, insights, or receive messages from the Arcturians. It is important to stay relaxed and receptive throughout the process, allowing the healing energy to flow freely.

Arcturian Energy Surgery is a powerful technique that can transform your life, promoting deep healing and the awakening of consciousness. By opening yourself to this experience, you will be connecting with the wisdom and unconditional love of the Arcturians, paving the way for a healthier, more balanced, and fulfilling life.

Chapter 6
Arcturian Crystals

Arcturian Crystals represent a direct bridge to higher energies, offering a path of healing and profound transformation. They are not just passive tools, but living entities acting in resonance with the highest frequencies of the universe. When interacting with these crystals, you connect to a unique vibration that harmonizes energy fields, unblocks old patterns of stagnation, and activates your highest potential. Their presence creates an environment of serenity and focus, allowing your energy to flow freely and promoting synergy between body, mind, and spirit. With each interaction, you access deeper levels of wisdom and light, awakening within yourself an expanded capacity for healing and expansion.

The crystalline energy of the Arcturians goes beyond simple material properties. These crystals emit frequencies that act directly on chakra alignment, activation of light codes stored in DNA, and elevation of consciousness to higher levels of perception. They are like conductors of universal energy, amplifying intentions and facilitating deep connections with spiritual realms. Through working with Arcturian Crystals, it is possible to unblock energy barriers, achieve deep meditative states, and access transformative insights that illuminate the path of spiritual evolution. Each crystal is a key that unlocks doors to dimensions of love, peace, and self-awareness.

In understanding and using Arcturian Crystals, you dive into a practice that unites energy science and spirituality. Their practical application, such as in meditations, sacred geometry grids, or even as protection amulets, brings tangible benefits to energetic and emotional health. More than that, they teach about the power of intention, showing that consciously directed energy has the power to manifest real and significant changes. Thus, when interacting with these crystals, you not only experience their healing effects but are also led to recognize your active role as a co-creator of your own energetic and spiritual reality.

Crystals are living beings that vibrate in harmony with the universe, emitting energy frequencies that can influence our energy field and promote well-being. The Arcturians, with their deep knowledge of crystalline energy, use specific crystals to amplify healing, activate light codes, and assist in the ascension process.

Crystals Used in Arcturian Healing: Arcturian Crystal: This crystal, of extraterrestrial origin, emanates a high vibration that facilitates connection with the Arcturians and multidimensional healing. Its energy promotes mental clarity, inner peace, and expansion of consciousness. Quartz: Quartz is a master crystal that amplifies energy and intention. It is used in conjunction with other crystals to enhance their effects and direct healing energy. Amethyst: Amethyst is a transmutation crystal that aids in releasing negative energies and emotional healing. It promotes inner peace, intuition, and spiritual connection. Rose Quartz: Rose quartz is the crystal of unconditional love and emotional healing. It opens the heart chakra, promoting compassion, forgiveness, and self-acceptance. Selenite: Selenite is a high-vibration crystal that purifies and elevates environmental energy. It facilitates connection with higher realms and channeling of healing energies. Citrine: Citrine is a crystal of prosperity and abundance that attracts positive energies and strengthens personal power. It increases vitality, creativity, and self-esteem. Fluorite: Fluorite is a crystal of mental clarity and concentration that aids in organizing thoughts and decision-making. It promotes mental harmony and inner peace.

Properties and Applications of Arcturian Crystals: Healing Amplification: Arcturian crystals amplify healing energy, enhancing the effects of Arcturian healing and other energy therapies. Light Code Activation: Arcturian crystals activate dormant light codes in DNA, awakening latent potentials and accelerating the ascension process. Chakra Harmonization: Crystals can be used to balance and harmonize chakras, promoting free flow of vital energy and physical, emotional, and spiritual well-being. Cleansing and Purification: Arcturian crystals purify the energy field, removing negative energies, blockages, and disease patterns. Energy Protection: Crystals create a protective shield around your energy field, protecting you from negative influences and dense energies. Consciousness Elevation: Arcturian crystals raise vibration and expand consciousness, facilitating connection with higher realms and spiritual awakening. Manifestation: Crystals can be programmed with specific intentions to manifest your desires and create the reality you wish.

How to Activate and Program Crystals:
1. Cleansing: Before using a crystal for the first time, it's important to cleanse it energetically to remove any residual energy. You can use running water, earth, incense, or selenite energy to cleanse your crystals.
2. Activation: To activate a crystal, hold it in your hands, connect with its energy, and visualize it being filled with light. You can also activate it using the energy of the sun, moon, or other crystals.
3. Programming: To program a crystal with a specific intention, hold it in your hands, focus on your desire, and visualize it manifesting. Express your intention aloud or mentally, imprinting your energy into the crystal.

How to Use Crystals in Arcturian Healing: Meditation: Hold the crystal in your hands during meditation to amplify connection with the Arcturians and receive their healing energies. Crystal Healing: Position crystals on chakras or body areas needing healing, visualizing energy flowing and promoting balance. Grid Creation: Create crystal grids with sacred geometry to amplify healing energy, harmonize the environment, and manifest your desires. Elixirs: Prepare crystal elixirs to ingest the healing energy of crystals and promote physical and energetic well-being. Amulets: Use crystals as protection and healing amulets, carrying them with you to receive their beneficial energies.

Working with Arcturian Crystals is more than using tools; it's an invitation to cultivate a deep relationship with the living and pulsating energy of the universe. Each crystal carries within itself a unique wisdom, a portal to higher dimensions that teach us about balance, intuition, and expansion. As we open ourselves to this interaction, we learn not only to receive their vibrations but also to channel our own energy more consciously and intentionally. Thus, Arcturian Crystals become luminous companions on our journey, reflecting the unlimited potential for transformation that dwells within each of us.

Chapter 7
Arcturian Symbols

Arcturian Symbols represent a vibrational language that connects directly with the higher dimensions, activating transformative energies and raising consciousness to cosmic levels. They are not just geometric shapes, but universal patterns of encoded energy, capable of unlocking dormant potentials and opening portals to a wisdom that transcends time and space. By interacting with these symbols, you are tuning into high frequencies that promote healing, balance, and alignment with the universal matrix. Each symbol is an expression of the divine, acting as a channel that integrates body, mind, and spirit in perfect harmony.

These symbols go beyond what the eyes can see, touching the deepest levels of our essence. Using Sacred Geometry as a basis, they resonate with the fundamental structure of the universe, connecting directly with the creative energy that permeates all things. When applied with intention, Arcturian symbols activate light codes in DNA, realigning the energy field and opening paths to new spiritual perceptions. This connection promotes a state of expanded presence, allowing you to access layers of wisdom that are often beyond mental comprehension, but which manifest as a sense of clarity, peace, and purpose.

By working with the Arcturian Symbols, you become a conscious co-creator of your energy reality. Whether through meditations, drawing symbols in sacred spaces, or using them as healing tools, the energy they bring manifests in a tangible way. They function as anchors of light, aligning your energy field with the higher dimensions and creating a bridge for connection with spiritual guides and universal wisdom. With continued use, you will notice an elevation in your vibration, an expansion of consciousness, and greater fluidity in the areas of your life that need balance and transformation.

Symbols are geometric shapes that carry specific meanings and energies. They act as keys that open portals to higher dimensions, activating light codes and awakening dormant potentials within our being. The Arcturians use sacred symbols in their healing and ascension work, transmitting high frequencies that promote harmonization and expansion of consciousness.

Sacred Geometry:

Sacred Geometry is the universal language of creation, a set of mathematical patterns and proportions that repeat in all life forms, from the structure of DNA to the formation of galaxies. Arcturian symbols are based on Sacred Geometry, expressing the harmony and divine order of the universe.

Arcturian Symbols and their Meanings:

- **Star of Arcturus:** Represents connection with Arcturian energy, multidimensional healing, and spiritual ascension. Activates light codes in DNA and promotes the expansion of consciousness.
- **Sacred Triangle:** Symbolizes the divine trinity, the union of body, mind, and spirit. Promotes harmony, balance, and energy protection.
- **Golden Spiral:** Represents the flow of vital energy, growth, and spiritual evolution. Activates the kundalini and facilitates connection with the Higher Self.
- **Flower of Life:** Symbolizes creation, the interconnection of all things, and the unity of the universe. Promotes harmony, healing, and expansion of consciousness.
- **Metatron's Cube:** Represents the matrix of creation, the sacred geometry that sustains all life forms. Promotes energy harmonization and connection with the higher realms.

- **Merkaba:** Symbolizes the vehicle of light that transports us to higher dimensions. Activates the personal Merkaba, facilitating astral travel and spiritual ascension.

How to Use Arcturian Symbols:
- **Meditation:** Visualize Arcturian symbols during meditation, allowing their energy to act on your energy field and promote healing and expansion of consciousness.
- **Healing:** Draw symbols on the body or on objects to direct healing energy and activate light codes.
- **Protection:** Use symbols as protective amulets, visualizing them around you to create an energy shield.
- **Harmonization of Environments:** Draw or place representations of symbols in environments to harmonize the energy of the place and promote well-being.
- **Creation of Mandalas:** Use Arcturian symbols in the creation of mandalas for meditation, healing, and spiritual elevation.

Activating the Symbols:
To activate the energy of Arcturian symbols, you can:
- **Visualize:** Clearly visualize the symbol, imagining it vibrant and radiant, emitting light and energy.
- **Draw:** Draw the symbol with your hands, focusing on its shape and meaning.
- **Mentalize:** Mentalize the symbol, repeating its name or associated mantra.
- **Use Crystals:** Place crystals on the symbol to amplify its energy.

Arcturian symbols are keys that open doors to healing, ascension, and connection with cosmic wisdom. By using the symbols with reverence and intention, you will be opening yourself to receive the healing energy and guidance of the Arcturians, expanding your consciousness and awakening your divine potential.

Chapter 8
Arcturian Meditation

Arcturian Meditation offers a deeply transformative experience, connecting you to the high energies of Arcturus and the unconditional love of its masters. This practice transcends traditional meditation by creating an energy portal that harmonizes your being on all levels, awakening the healing power and spiritual potential that resides within you. With each breath, you are enveloped by a vibrant light that cleanses, heals, and uplifts, allowing you to access a state of inner peace and cosmic connection. Through this process, your consciousness expands, and you align with universal wisdom and the true essence of who you are.

The practice uses powerful tools such as the activation of the Threefold Flame, a symbol of the divine triad of wisdom, love, and power that resides in your heart. By visualizing the blue, gold, and pink flames expanding within you, it is possible to access deep levels of transformation. This aligned energy state not only promotes emotional and spiritual healing, but also facilitates clear insights into your life journey, revealing ways to overcome challenges and manifest your highest purpose. Each stage of meditation is designed to guide you to a state of communion with the cosmos, while strengthening your energy and vibrational field.

By integrating Arcturian Meditation into your routine, you will be cultivating a sacred space within yourself, where healing and growth become constant. Regular practice strengthens your connection with the Arcturians, allowing you to receive their messages and healing energies more easily. This experience empowers you to release energy blocks, transform limiting patterns, and access a higher vibration. At the same time, it invites you to explore your divine essence, helping you to align with the natural flow of life and walk in harmony with the universal light.

Meditation is an ancient practice that calms the mind, harmonizes emotions, and connects us with our divine essence. Arcturian Meditation goes further, opening a portal to connect with the beings of light from Arcturus, allowing you to receive their healing energies, their wisdom, and their unconditional love. It is an opportunity to connect with your own divinity, awakening the Threefold Flame — the flame of wisdom, love, and power — that resides in your heart.

Preparing for Meditation:
1. **Find a quiet place:** Choose a quiet place free from distractions where you can sit or lie down comfortably.
2. **Purify the environment:** Use incense, crystals, or other methods to purify the environment and create a sacred atmosphere.
3. **Connect with your heart:** Breathe deeply and focus your attention on your heart, the center of love and compassion.
4. **Invoke the Arcturians:** With reverence and gratitude, invoke the presence of the Arcturians, requesting their assistance and guidance during meditation.

Step by Step Arcturian Meditation:
1. **Relaxation:** Sit or lie down comfortably, close your eyes, and relax your body. Breathe deeply, observing the air entering and leaving your lungs.
2. **Visualization:** Imagine a portal of light opening above your head, connecting you with the energy of Arcturus. Visualize a golden light descending from the portal and enveloping your body, filling you with peace and serenity.
3. **Connection with Arcturus:** Feel the loving energy of the Arcturians flowing through you, harmonizing your chakras and raising your vibration. Allow yourself to be enveloped by this energy, feeling the peace and serenity that emanate from Arcturus.

4. **Activating the Threefold Flame:** Visualize a threefold flame — blue, gold, and pink — igniting in your heart. Feel the flame of wisdom, love, and power expanding within your being, filling you with light and strength.
5. **Communication with the Arcturians:** Open yourself to receive messages from the Arcturians. They can come in the form of images, thoughts, feelings, or intuitions. Trust your inner wisdom and allow yourself to be guided.
6. **Healing and Transformation:** Allow Arcturian energy to act on your being, promoting physical, emotional, mental, and spiritual healing. Visualize energy removing blockages, healing wounds, and restoring balance on all levels.
7. **Gratitude:** Thank the Arcturians for their presence and assistance during meditation. Also thank yourself for dedicating yourself to this practice and for opening yourself to healing and transformation.
8. **Return:** When you feel ready, bring your attention back to your body and your surroundings. Take a deep breath and open your eyes slowly.

Tips for Deepening Meditation:
- **Regular practice:** Meditation is like a muscle that needs to be exercised. Practice Arcturian Meditation regularly to strengthen your connection with the Arcturians and deepen your experience.
- **Music:** Use soft, relaxing music to create an atmosphere conducive to meditation.
- **Aromas:** Use essential oils with calming and relaxing properties, such as lavender and chamomile.
- **Crystals:** Use crystals that aid in meditation and connection with the Arcturians, such as amethyst, rose quartz, and selenite.
- **Intention:** Set a clear intention for your meditation, be it healing, relaxation, connection with the Arcturians, or expansion of consciousness.

Benefits of Arcturian Meditation:

- **Connection with the Arcturians:** Strengthens the connection with the Arcturians, allowing you to receive their healing energies, their wisdom, and their unconditional love.
- **Multidimensional Healing:** Promotes physical, emotional, mental, and spiritual healing, harmonizing your energy fields and restoring balance.
- **Expansion of Consciousness:** Raises your vibration and expands your consciousness, opening the way for spiritual awakening and ascension.
- **Inner Peace:** Calms the mind, reduces stress and anxiety, promoting inner peace and emotional well-being.
- **Self-knowledge:** Facilitates the process of self-knowledge, helping in understanding your patterns, beliefs, and emotions.
- **Awakening of the Threefold Flame:** Activates the Threefold Flame in your heart, awakening the wisdom, love, and power that reside within your being.

Arcturian Meditation is a journey into your inner self, an opportunity to connect with the divine source and experience the deep peace and wisdom that emanate from Arcturus. By dedicating yourself to this practice, you will be opening the doors to healing, transformation, and ascension, treading a path of light towards your true essence.

Chapter 9
Conscious Breathing

Conscious Breathing is a powerful bridge between your physical essence and your spiritual dimension, connecting you with the universal source of vital energy. Through it, you can unlock energy flows, dissolve emotional tensions, and realign your being with higher states of balance and harmony. Each conscious breath becomes a moment of healing and transformation, allowing prana - the vital energy that permeates the universe - to flow freely and regeneratively in your body. This practice is not just a technique, but a portal to access inner peace, activate your energy centers, and expand your consciousness.

By immersing yourself in Arcturian breathing techniques, you discover that breathing is not just a physical act, but a sacred tool for self-connection and self-healing. Visualizing prana filling your being with light during inhalation and releasing stagnant energies on exhalation creates a continuous cycle of energy renewal. In addition, practices such as Threefold Flame Breathing go beyond relaxation, allowing you to access deeper aspects of your divine essence. The activation of the blue, gold, and pink flames in your heart awakens wisdom, love, and power, creating a vibrational field that harmonizes your being on all levels.

With regular practice of Conscious Breathing, you can transform the way you interact with your body and your energy. It not only helps to calm the mind and reduce stress, but also puts you in tune with higher frequencies, facilitating connection with the Arcturians and your own inner wisdom. By dedicating a few minutes a day to this practice, you will discover a new vitality and clarity, strengthening your ability to navigate life's challenges with serenity and purpose. Take a deep breath, let vital energy permeate every aspect of your existence, and feel the transformative power this practice can bring to your journey.

Breathing is the basis of life, a vital process that sustains our physical body and profoundly influences our emotional and mental state. The Arcturians, masters in the art of energy healing, recognize breathing as a powerful tool to balance energies, release blocked emotions, and access higher states of consciousness. Through Conscious Breathing, you can connect with the vital energy of the universe, harmonize your chakras, and awaken inner healing.

The Influence of Breathing on Vital Energy:
Breathing is the key to the flow of vital energy (prana) in our body. When we breathe deeply and consciously, we allow prana to flow freely, nourishing every cell and revitalizing our being. On the other hand, shallow and irregular breathing can block the flow of energy, generating imbalances and affecting physical, emotional, and mental health.

Arcturian Breathing Techniques:
- **Arcturian Activation Breathing:** This technique uses visualization and deep breathing to activate the chakras and energize the body. Inhale deeply visualizing pranic energy entering your lungs and filling every cell in your body with light. Exhale slowly, releasing any tension or negative energy.
- **Threefold Flame Breathing:** This technique uses visualization and breathing to activate the Threefold Flame in the heart. Breathe in visualizing the blue flame of wisdom expanding in your mind. Breathe out visualizing the golden flame of love filling your heart. Inhale again visualizing the pink flame of power strengthening your body. Repeat the cycle several times, feeling the Threefold Flame intensify within your being.
- **Healing Breath:** This technique uses breath and intention to direct healing energy to specific areas of the body. Inhale deeply, visualizing pranic energy entering your

lungs and focusing on the area that needs healing. Exhale slowly, visualizing healing energy flowing to that area and promoting regeneration.
- **Connection Breathing:** This technique uses breathing and visualization to connect with the energy of Arcturus. Inhale deeply, visualizing a portal of light opening above your head and Arcturian energy descending and enveloping your body. Exhale slowly, feeling the connection with the Arcturians grow stronger.

Conscious Breathing Practice:
1. **Find a quiet place:** Choose a quiet place free from distractions where you can sit or lie down comfortably.
2. **Posture:** Keep your spine straight and your body relaxed.
3. **Concentration:** Focus your attention on your breathing, observing the air entering and leaving your lungs.
4. **Deep breathing:** Breathe deeply, expanding your abdomen on inhalation and contracting it on exhalation.
5. **Rhythm:** Find a breathing rhythm that is comfortable for you.
6. **Visualization:** Use visualization to enhance the effects of breathing, imagining pranic energy flowing through your body and promoting healing and balance.
7. **Intention:** Set a clear intention for your breathing practice, be it healing, relaxation, connection with the Arcturians, or expansion of consciousness.

Benefits of Conscious Breathing:
- **Healing:** Promotes physical, emotional, and mental healing, releasing energy blocks and restoring balance.
- **Relaxation:** Reduces stress, anxiety, and muscle tension, promoting deep relaxation and inner peace.
- **Energy:** Increases vitality and energy, revitalizing body and mind.
- **Connection:** Strengthens the connection with the Higher Self, spirit guides, and the energy of Arcturus.
- **Awareness:** Expands awareness, increases intuition, and facilitates access to higher states of perception.

- **Balance:** Harmonizes the chakras and balances the subtle bodies, promoting integral well-being.

Conscious Breathing is a powerful tool that is always available to you. By mastering Arcturian breathing techniques, you can access a state of healing, balance, and deep connection with cosmic wisdom. Take a deep breath, connect with your breath, and allow vital energy to flow freely, awakening your inner potential and guiding you on your journey of ascension.

Chapter 10
Healing Sounds

Healing Sounds represent a unique vibrational path to access universal harmony and activate profound processes of healing and transformation. Each sound, note, or vibration interacts directly with the energy field, creating an impact that goes beyond the physical and resonates on emotional, mental, and spiritual levels. This sonic interaction can release energy blocks, balance disharmonious frequencies, and revitalize the connection with the vital energy of the universe. More than a sensory experience, healing sounds are portals to elevated states of consciousness and a deep alignment with your divine essence.

Healing through sound utilizes the body's natural ability to resonate with harmonic vibrations. When exposed to sacred mantras, carefully composed music, or the serene sounds of nature, the energy field is rebalanced, and the chakras align, allowing energy to flow freely and restoratively. The Arcturians, with their advanced wisdom, use specific frequencies that act directly on DNA, activating dormant light codes and promoting a transformation that extends to body, mind, and spirit. These sounds also create an inner space of peace and clarity, allowing a deeper connection with the higher realms.

Integrating Healing Sounds into your life is a way to align yourself with the natural flow of the universe. Whether listening to mantras with intention, using instruments like crystal bowls, or connecting with the sounds of nature, you can access states of relaxation and expanded consciousness. This practice not only promotes healing and well-being but also awakens within you an expanded perception of interconnectedness with the cosmos.

Allowing sound vibrations to fill your being is a way to open doors to energy renewal and greater alignment with your highest purpose.

The Arcturians, masters of the art of vibrational healing, understand the power of sound as a tool for transformation. They use specific sound frequencies to harmonize the subtle bodies, awaken dormant potentials, and promote healing on deep levels. Through Healing Sounds, you can connect with the harmony of the universe, release patterns of disease, and activate light codes in your DNA.

The Influence of Sound on the Energy Field:

Sound is vibration, and everything in the universe vibrates at a specific frequency. Our physical body and our subtle bodies also have vibrational frequencies, and when these frequencies resonate with harmonious sounds, a process of harmonization and healing occurs. On the other hand, dissonant sounds can generate disharmony and negatively affect our energy field.

Healing Sounds in Arcturian Healing:
- **Mantras:** Mantras are sacred words or phrases that, when chanted with intention, emit vibrations that promote healing, protection, and spiritual elevation. The Arcturians use specific mantras to activate light codes, harmonize the chakras, and connect with the energy of Arcturus.
- **Music:** Music is a universal language that transcends the barriers of verbal language, touching the soul and promoting healing on deep levels. The Arcturians use specific melodies and harmonies to balance energies, calm the mind, and awaken positive emotions.
- **Sounds of Nature:** The sounds of nature, such as birdsong, the sound of ocean waves, and the murmur of the wind, have harmonious frequencies that promote relaxation, healing, and connection with the vital energy of the Earth.
- **Arcturian Frequencies:** The Arcturians use specific sound frequencies to activate multidimensional healing, awaken consciousness, and accelerate the ascension

process. These frequencies can be transmitted through Arcturian technologies, such as healing chambers, or channeled by therapists who work with Arcturian energy.

How to Use Healing Sounds:
- **Listen with Intention:** When listening to mantras, music, or sounds of nature, focus on the intention of healing and harmonization. Visualize the sound vibrations penetrating your being, removing blockages and restoring balance.
- **Chant Mantras:** Chant Arcturian mantras with reverence and concentration, feeling the sound vibrations resonating in your body and raising your vibration.
- **Play Instruments:** Playing musical instruments, such as crystal bowls, Tibetan bells, and flutes, can generate harmonious frequencies that promote healing and relaxation.
- **Sing:** Singing is a powerful way to express emotions, release blocked energies, and connect with your divine essence.
- **Dance:** Dancing to music that raises your vibration promotes the release of tension, the expression of creativity, and connection with joy.

Benefits of Healing Sounds:
- **Healing:** Promotes physical, emotional, and mental healing, harmonizing energies and restoring balance.
- **Relaxation:** Reduces stress, anxiety, and muscle tension, promoting deep relaxation and inner peace.
- **Raising Vibration:** Raises vibration, facilitating connection with the higher realms and the energy of Arcturus.
- **Expansion of Consciousness:** Expands consciousness, increases intuition, and facilitates access to higher states of perception.
- **DNA Activation:** Activates dormant light codes in DNA, awakening latent potentials and accelerating the ascension process.

- **Harmonization of the Chakras:** Balances and harmonizes the chakras, promoting the free flow of vital energy.

Healing Sounds are a gift from the universe, a powerful tool for healing, transformation, and ascension. By opening yourself to the sound experience, you will be connecting with cosmic harmony and awakening inner healing. Vibrate in tune with the universe, allowing healing sounds to guide you on your journey of evolution and expansion of consciousness.

Chapter 11
Arcturian Chromotherapy

Arcturian Chromotherapy emerges as a vibrant and deeply transformative practice, based on the interaction between colors and the human energy field. Colors, each with its specific frequency, carry properties that directly influence the chakras, promoting balance, vitality, and spiritual connection. This method, brought by Arcturian wisdom, not only resonates with physical healing but also acts on the emotional and spiritual dimensions, leading to a full integration of being. By immersing yourself in this practice, you discover how to channel the energy of colors to align and strengthen the energetic essence of each individual, opening paths to self-knowledge and transcendence.

Each hue used in Arcturian Chromotherapy plays a unique role. Red, for example, is a color that radiates strength and vitality, ideal for activating the root chakra and strengthening the connection with the Earth. Orange brings out creativity and joy, harmonizing the sacral chakra and awakening the pleasure of living. Shades of yellow are allies in increasing personal power and mental clarity, balancing the solar plexus. Green, with its energy of healing and harmony, aligns with the heart chakra, promoting unconditional love and emotional balance. Shades of blue and indigo act to open channels of communication and perception, connecting the individual to their deepest intuitions, while violet elevates spirituality, uniting the crown chakra to the divine source. This approach integrates not only the symbolism of colors but also their practical applications in techniques ranging from meditative visualizations to the use of crystals and specific lights.

By exploring the therapeutic application of colors, one discovers that Arcturian Chromotherapy transcends a purely technical approach, assuming a role of reconnection with inner wisdom. It is a journey that combines intuition, intention, and energy science. Practicing this technique is not limited to harmonizing momentary imbalances but expands to build a solid foundation of continuous well-being. Whether through meditation, the conscious consumption of colorful foods, or the choice of clothes and objects that resonate with the necessary frequency, each act is transformed into a healing ritual. Thus, by embracing the vibrational spectrum of colors as a tool for transformation, space is opened for a more enlightened, harmonious life full of integral well-being.

The Arcturians, masters of the art of vibrational healing, understand the profound influence of colors on our energy field. Each color has a specific vibratory frequency that resonates with our chakras and subtle bodies, promoting harmonization and balance. Through Arcturian Chromotherapy, you can use colors as instruments of healing, awakening the inner healing power and promoting well-being at all levels of your being.

Therapeutic Properties of Colors:
- **Red:** Energy, vitality, strength, courage, passion. Stimulates the root chakra, blood circulation, and physical strength.
- **Orange:** Creativity, joy, enthusiasm, sexuality, self-esteem. Stimulates the sacral chakra, digestion, and vitality.
- **Yellow:** Intelligence, concentration, learning, mental clarity, personal power. Stimulates the solar plexus chakra, nervous system, and self-esteem.
- **Green:** Healing, balance, harmony, unconditional love, compassion. Stimulates the heart chakra, immune system, and emotional balance.
- **Blue:** Communication, expression, inner peace, tranquility, intuition. Stimulates the throat chakra, communication, and creative expression.

- **Indigo:** Intuition, wisdom, perception, inner vision, spiritual connection. Stimulates the brow chakra, intuition, and connection with the Higher Self.
- **Violet:** Spirituality, transmutation, purification, elevation, connection with the divine. Stimulates the crown chakra, spirituality, and connection with the divine source.

Techniques for Applying Arcturian Chromotherapy:
- **Visualization:** Visualize the color you want to use surrounding your body or the chakra that needs to be harmonized. Imagine the color penetrating your being, promoting healing and balance.
- **Meditation with Colors:** Meditate by visualizing the color you want to work with, feeling its vibration and allowing it to act on your energy field.
- **Light Baths:** Use colored lamps or light projectors to bathe your body with the color you need.
- **Crystals:** Use crystals of the color you want to work with to amplify the healing energy and direct it to the chakra or area of the body that needs to be harmonized.
- **Clothes and Objects:** Use clothes, accessories, and objects of the color you want to work with to receive their healing vibrations.
- **Foods:** Consume foods of the color you want to work with to absorb their energies and promote well-being.

Applying Chromotherapy to the Chakras:
- **Root Chakra (Red):** Use red to strengthen the root chakra, increasing vitality, physical energy, and connection to the Earth.
- **Sacral Chakra (Orange):** Use orange to harmonize the sacral chakra, awakening creativity, joy, and sexuality.
- **Solar Plexus Chakra (Yellow):** Use yellow to balance the solar plexus chakra, increasing personal power, self-esteem, and mental clarity.
- **Heart Chakra (Green):** Use green to heal the heart chakra, promoting unconditional love, compassion, and emotional balance.

- **Throat Chakra (Blue):** Use blue to harmonize the throat chakra, improving communication, expression, and creativity.
- **Brow Chakra (Indigo):** Use indigo to activate the brow chakra, awakening intuition, wisdom, and connection with the Higher Self.
- **Crown Chakra (Violet):** Use violet to raise the vibration of the crown chakra, strengthening spirituality and connection with the divine source.

Benefits of Arcturian Chromotherapy:
- **Healing:** Promotes physical, emotional, and mental healing, harmonizing energies and restoring balance.
- **Energy Balance:** Balances the chakras and subtle bodies, promoting the free flow of vital energy.
- **Raising Vibration:** Raises vibration, facilitating connection with the higher realms and the energy of Arcturus.
- **Well-being:** Promotes physical, emotional, and spiritual well-being, increasing vitality, inner peace, and joy of living.
- **Self-knowledge:** Assists in the process of self-knowledge, allowing you to understand the energy needs of your body and mind.

Arcturian Chromotherapy is a powerful tool for healing and transformation. By using colors wisely and intentionally, you can harmonize your chakras, balance your energies, and awaken inner healing. Allow the vibrant colors of the rainbow to guide you on your journey of ascension, filling your life with light, harmony, and well-being.

Chapter 12
DNA Activation

DNA Activation is a transformative process that invites you to explore the depths of your existence and rediscover your unlimited potential. More than a set of genetic codes, human DNA is a multidimensional portal that holds the records of your divine essence and higher abilities. This technique, based on Arcturian wisdom, awakens the dormant strands of DNA, allowing access to expanded levels of consciousness and latent abilities that transcend conventional human limitations. By activating these structures, you begin a journey of healing, connection, and evolution that resonates in all dimensions of your being.

At the core of this process is the understanding that DNA has 12 strands, of which only two are active in most people. The "dormant" strands, often called "junk" DNA by conventional science, contain light codes that reflect our divine potential. The activation of these strands is carried out through specific vibrational frequencies, facilitated by Arcturian energy, which resonate with the human energy field to release these codes. As these frequencies activate the records in DNA, an expansion of consciousness occurs, which enables everything from physical healing to the awakening of abilities such as intuition, telepathy, and direct spiritual connection.

The benefits of this activation are broad and deeply impactful. In addition to stimulating cellular rejuvenation and strengthening the immune system, it promotes a state of balance and inner peace, while facilitating the manifestation of dreams and desires aligned with your highest essence. Creativity is amplified, as is the ability to understand and navigate between higher dimensions of reality. Through the strengthened connection with the Higher Self and spiritual guides, life takes on a new purpose, marked by clarity, harmony, and inspiration.

This process is not limited to activation itself, but also requires a period of integration, in which the body, mind, and spirit adjust to the new frequencies. During this phase, practices such as meditation, healthy eating, creative expression, and connection with nature are fundamental to consolidating the changes. Over time, these transformations manifest in the form of a more balanced, abundant life full of possibilities. Arcturian DNA Activation is, therefore, a call to embrace your true essence and access the unlimited power that resides within you.

The Arcturians, with their deep knowledge of genetics and multidimensional energy, teach us that human DNA is much more than just a genetic code. It is a portal to our divine essence, an archive that contains information about our history, our abilities, and our unlimited potential. Through Arcturian DNA Activation, you can awaken these dormant potentials, expanding your consciousness, accessing higher abilities, and accelerating your journey of ascension.

Multidimensional DNA:

Human DNA has 12 strands, with only 2 active in most people. The other 10 strands, known as "junk" DNA, contain dormant light codes waiting to be activated. Arcturian DNA Activation uses specific energy frequencies to awaken these strands, releasing information and abilities that were blocked.

Benefits of DNA Activation:
- **Expansion of Consciousness:** DNA activation expands your consciousness, allowing you to access higher dimensions of reality and understand the interconnectedness of all things.
- **Healing:** Activates the body's natural healing process, strengthening the immune system and promoting cellular regeneration.

- **Intuition and Psychic Abilities:** Awakens intuition, clairvoyance, telepathy, and other psychic abilities.
- **Spiritual Connection:** Strengthens the connection with the Higher Self, spiritual guides, and the divine source.
- **Rejuvenation:** Slows down the aging process and promotes longevity.
- **Creativity:** Increases creativity, inspiration, and the ability to manifest your dreams.
- **Inner Peace:** Promotes inner peace, emotional balance, and harmony in your life.

Stages of DNA Activation:
1. **Preparation:** Prepare for DNA activation through meditation, conscious breathing, and connection with Arcturian energy.
2. **Intention:** Clearly define your intention for DNA activation, visualizing the results you want to achieve.
3. **Invocation:** Invoke the presence of the Arcturians and ask for their assistance in activating your DNA.
4. **Arcturian Frequencies:** The Arcturians use sound, light, and vibrational frequencies to activate the dormant strands of your DNA. Visualize these frequencies penetrating your being, awakening light codes and activating your divine potential.
5. **Integration:** After activation, take time to integrate the new frequencies, allowing your body and mind to adjust to the changes.

Integrating the New Frequencies:

After DNA Activation, it is important to integrate the new frequencies into your being, allowing them to manifest in your life. Some tips for integrating the new frequencies:
- **Meditation:** Meditate regularly to connect with your Higher Self and integrate the new energies.
- **Self-care:** Take care of your physical body through a healthy diet, exercise, and adequate rest.
- **Creative Expression:** Express your creativity through art, music, writing, or other forms of expression.

- **Connection with Nature:** Spend time in nature to connect with the vital energy of the Earth and integrate the new frequencies.
- **Gratitude:** Cultivate gratitude for all the blessings in your life and for the new opportunities that open up for you.

Awakening your Divine Potential:

Arcturian DNA Activation is a gift from the Arcturians to humanity, an opportunity to awaken our divine potential and manifest our true essence. By activating your DNA, you will be opening the doors to a new reality, where healing, abundance, inner peace, and connection with the divine become a reality in your life. Trust in the wisdom of the Arcturians, surrender to the activation process, and allow your being to be illuminated with the light of your own divinity.

Chapter 13
Healing the Past

Healing the past represents a transformative opportunity for liberation, allowing you to reconnect with your true essence and live fully in the present. Through the loving and intuitive approach of the Arcturians, this practice delves into the depths of your being to access memories, traumas, and crystallized patterns that still influence your current life. More than confronting the past, it is about reframing it with compassion, transmuting dense energies into learning and inner strength. This journey of self-transformation not only releases the weight of past experiences but also opens space for you to flourish with lightness and authenticity.

Throughout life, painful experiences and limiting beliefs leave impressions on the energy field, shaping behavioral patterns that often repeat unconsciously. Arcturian Past Healing allows you to identify and understand these hidden influences, providing clarity about their origins and helping to dissolve them. Guided by Arcturian wisdom, you are encouraged to revisit these experiences with a compassionate eye, perceiving them as chapters that contributed to your growth journey, not as chains that bind you. This process promotes a balanced integration between the past and the present, allowing you to regain control over your personal narrative.

The techniques involved are profoundly effective and encompass practices such as regression, forgiveness, and reframing. Regression, for example, allows you to access deep memories, whether from childhood or past lives, enabling you to identify and release blocked energies. Forgiveness, both of yourself and others, dissolves emotional bonds, replacing hurt with a state of peace and compassion. By reframing traumatic events, you transform your perceptions, recognizing the learning and strength gained through these experiences. In addition, working with karmic release and inner child healing helps to undo negative cycles, harmonize the present, and create a solid foundation for a lighter and more enlightened future.

This healing journey is not just a process of liberation, but also an opportunity to reconnect with your highest essence. By leaving behind the shadows of the past, you strengthen your ability to live authentically, embracing the fullness of the present moment. It is in this state of presence that true transformation occurs, allowing joy, love, and abundance to flow freely in your life. Under the guidance of the Arcturians, you discover that the past, instead of a burden, can become a springboard for your evolution and for the manifestation of a reality full of harmony and purpose.

The past, although already vanished in time, can leave deep marks on our being. Traumatic experiences, painful relationships, dysfunctional family patterns, and limiting beliefs can take root in our subconscious, affecting our health, our relationships, and our ability to be happy in the present. Arcturian Past Healing invites us to revisit these experiences with compassion and wisdom, releasing blocked energies and reframing the past so that it becomes a springboard for growth and evolution.

Understanding the Influence of the Past:

The past shapes who we are today, but it doesn't have to define us. The experiences we live, the emotions we feel, and the beliefs we form throughout life crystallize in our energy field, creating patterns that repeat and prevent us from moving forward. Arcturian Past Healing helps us identify these patterns, understand their origins, and release blocked energies, allowing healing and transformation to occur.

Arcturian Past Healing Techniques:
- **Regression:** Regression, guided by the Arcturians, allows you to access memories, whether from this life or past lives, to reframe experiences and release blocked emotions. Through regression, you can understand the origin of repetitive patterns, traumas, and blockages, bringing light and healing to the wounds of the past.
- **Forgiveness:** Forgiveness is a powerful key to healing the past. Forgiving yourself and others for past hurts and pains releases the dense energies that bind you to suffering, opening space for inner peace and freedom. The Arcturians guide you in this process, helping you to cultivate compassion and unconditional love.
- **Reframing:** Reframing is the process of giving new meaning to past experiences, transforming them into learning and opportunities for growth. By reframing the past, you free yourself from the bonds of suffering and empower yourself to create a more positive and happy future.
- **Karmic Release:** Karma is the law of cause and effect that governs the universe. Past actions, whether positive or negative, generate consequences that manifest in our present life. Arcturian Past Healing assists in the release of negative karmas, harmonizing energies and paving the way for a lighter and more balanced future.
- **Inner Child Healing:** Arcturian Past Healing also focuses on healing the inner child, that part of us that carries the wounds and traumas of childhood. By healing the inner child, you free yourself from patterns of abandonment, rejection, and insecurity, reconnecting with joy, spontaneity, and unconditional love.

Applying Past Healing:
1. **Preparation:** Prepare for past healing by creating a sacred space, connecting with your heart, and invoking the presence of the Arcturians.

2. **Intention:** Clearly define your intention for past healing, specifying the areas you want to work on and the results you want to achieve.
3. **Techniques:** Use the Arcturian Past Healing techniques that resonate with you, such as regression, forgiveness, reframing, and karmic release.
4. **Visualization:** Use visualization to connect with memories, sending light and healing to the situations and people involved.
5. **Emotions:** Allow yourself to feel the emotions that arise during the healing process, without judgment or resistance. The Arcturians will help you to embrace and release these emotions with love and compassion.
6. **Integration:** After healing the past, take time to integrate the new energies, allowing the healing to manifest in your present life.

Freeing Yourself from the Past to Live the Present:

Arcturian Past Healing is an invitation to free yourself from the bonds of the past and walk a path of lightness, healing, and fullness in the present. By reframing your experiences, freeing yourself from karmas, and healing the wounds of the past, you open space for a radiant future where joy, love, and abundance flow freely. Trust in the wisdom of the Arcturians, surrender to the healing process, and allow the past to become a springboard for your evolution and ascension.

Chapter 14
Healing the Present

Healing the Present is a practice that calls us to live fully in the now, recognizing the transformative power contained in each moment. It is in the present that choices gain meaning, that challenges become teachers, and that life reveals itself in its entirety. Under the loving guidance of the Arcturians, this technique promotes the release of reactive and conditioned patterns, replacing them with conscious and balanced actions. By cultivating a full presence, you discover that the present is not just a passing moment, but a portal to healing, learning, and creating a reality more aligned with your essence.

Being present requires mindfulness, a practice of observing thoughts, emotions, and sensations without judgment or attachment. In this state, you begin to identify the internal narratives and patterns that shape your choices. Instead of reacting impulsively, you learn to respond in a balanced way, transforming even the most difficult challenges into opportunities for growth. The Arcturians teach that by anchoring yourself in the now, you harmonize not only your emotional state but also your energy field, promoting well-being and clarity on all levels.

The practice of Healing the Present encompasses techniques that strengthen the connection with the present moment. Mindfulness, conscious breathing, and welcoming emotions are essential steps to balance the body and mind. Simultaneously, conscious communication and intentional manifestation allow you to build more authentic relationships and attract situations aligned with your highest goals. This process is not just about solving problems, but about building a more harmonious and rewarding life, where each moment is valued as an essential part of your journey.

By adopting Healing the Present as a continuous practice, you empower yourself to live with gratitude and presence, creating a state of balance and serenity. Life's challenges, instead of sources of suffering, become opportunities for learning and self-transformation. In this way, you navigate through existence with clarity and purpose, discovering that the present is the place where your fullness can flourish. Under the light and wisdom of the Arcturians, you are invited to embrace the now as the greatest gift life can offer.

While Healing the Past frees us from the bonds that bind us to suffering, Healing the Present invites us to be fully present in the here and now, transforming each moment into an opportunity for growth, healing, and expansion. It is in the present that life happens, and it is in it that we can create the reality we desire, free from the pains of the past and worries about the future. Arcturian Present Healing teaches us to embrace each moment with gratitude, transforming challenges into opportunities and cultivating inner peace amidst life's turbulences.

Awakening to the Present:

In our fast-paced society, it is common to get lost in thoughts about the past or worries about the future, disconnecting from the present moment. Arcturian Present Healing invites us to awaken to the now, cultivating mindfulness and awareness of every thought, emotion, and sensation that arises in our being. By being present, we become able to observe our patterns, make conscious choices, and create the reality we desire.

Arcturian Present Healing Techniques:

- **Mindfulness:** Mindfulness is the practice of being present in every moment, observing your thoughts, emotions, and sensations without judgment. By cultivating mindfulness, you become more aware of your reactive patterns, allowing you to choose how to respond to challenges in a more balanced and conscious way.

- **Emotional Management:** Emotions are energies in motion that profoundly influence our health and well-being. Arcturian Present Healing teaches us to recognize, embrace, and manage our emotions in a healthy way, transforming them into allies in our growth journey.
- **Energy Healing:** The Arcturians use energy healing techniques to harmonize your chakras, balance your subtle bodies, and dissolve negative energy patterns that may be affecting your health and well-being in the present.
- **Conscious Communication:** Conscious communication is the key to healthy and harmonious relationships. The Arcturians teach us to communicate our needs and emotions clearly, respectfully, and assertively, creating deeper and more authentic connections.
- **Manifestation:** Arcturian Present Healing empowers us to manifest the reality we desire, using the law of attraction and the power of intention. By vibrating at the frequency of what we desire, we attract into our lives experiences, people, and situations that resonate with our dreams and aspirations.

Applying Present Healing:

1. **Presence:** Cultivate presence in the present moment through mindfulness, observing your thoughts, emotions, and sensations without judgment.
2. **Breathing:** Use conscious breathing to anchor yourself in the present and calm the mind.
3. **Acceptance:** Embrace your emotions with compassion, without trying to repress or control them. Allow yourself to feel and observe your emotions without judgment.
4. **Expression:** Express your emotions in a healthy way, whether through writing, art, dialogue, or other forms of creative expression.
5. **Boundaries:** Set healthy boundaries in your relationships, communicating your needs and expectations clearly and respectfully.

6. **Gratitude:** Cultivate gratitude for the blessings in your life, appreciating each moment and recognizing the abundance that surrounds you.

Creating a Conscious and Balanced Present:

Arcturian Present Healing invites us to live with awareness, presence, and gratitude, transforming each moment into an opportunity for healing, growth, and expansion. By mastering the techniques of Present Healing, you become able to navigate the waters of life with serenity and clarity, creating a harmonious, happy, and abundant present. Trust in the wisdom of the Arcturians, surrender to the flow of life, and allow the healing energy of the present to guide you on your journey of ascension.

Chapter 15
Healing the Future

Healing the Future is a powerful practice that empowers you to consciously shape tomorrow, transforming your intentions and dreams into concrete realities. This Arcturian approach offers an expansive view of time, where the future is perceived as a field of infinite possibilities, waiting to be shaped by your creative energy and focus. More than a technique, it is an invitation to abandon fears, limiting beliefs, and negative expectations, replacing them with clarity, confidence, and conscious action. Through this practice, you become the architect of your own destiny, aligning your choices with your highest purpose.

Building a radiant future begins with releasing emotional and mental blocks that often condition our expectations. Fears of the unknown and traumas of the past can cast shadows over tomorrow, creating invisible barriers that limit the potential for creation. Arcturian Future Healing teaches that by reprogramming these perceptions and cultivating a clear and optimistic vision, you access a state of flow that attracts circumstances and opportunities aligned with your desires. It is in this moment of clarity that visualization becomes a transformative tool, allowing you to experience, in your mind and heart, the reality you wish to create, while sending this energy to the universe.

This practice is strengthened by the use of clear intentions and affirmations. Setting specific intentions for the future is like planting seeds in the fertile soil of your consciousness. Nourishing them with positive affirmations and consistent actions ensures that these seeds grow and flourish. Co-creation, one of the pillars of this technique, reminds you that you are not alone in the manifestation process; there is a constant dance between your individual energy and the universal forces that work in harmony to materialize your aspirations. Trusting this flow and aligning your actions with your intuition allows the path to unfold naturally and fluidly.

Healing the Future is not just about designing a destiny, but also about living with presence and purpose. Each step taken today directly reflects the future you are building. When you connect with the Arcturians and use the tools of visualization, intention, and release of fears, a space opens for the future to be not only imagined, but experienced in its most authentic and abundant form. Thus, by adopting this practice, you transform the future into a vibrant extension of the present, where dreams become reality and where confidence in yourself and the universe is the foundation of your journey.

Healing the Future is not about predicting what will happen, but about creating the future you desire. It is an invitation to free yourself from limiting expectations, fears, and uncertainties that prevent you from dreaming big and building a prosperous and happy future. The Arcturians, with their expanded vision of time and space, teach us that the future is a field of infinite possibilities, and that we are co-creators of our reality. Through Arcturian Future Healing, you can connect with your inner power, define your intentions, and manifest the future you desire.

Freeing Yourself from Expectations:
Often, we carry limiting expectations about the future, based on past experiences, fears, and negative beliefs. These expectations can prevent us from dreaming big and creating a future that truly inspires us. Arcturian Future Healing invites us to free ourselves from these expectations, opening space for a future of infinite possibilities.

Arcturian Future Healing Techniques:
- **Visualization:** Visualization is a powerful tool for creating the future you desire. Imagine yourself living the future you desire, feeling the emotions, sensations, and experiences as if they were already happening.

Visualization sends a clear signal to the universe, attracting into your life the people, situations, and opportunities that resonate with your dreams.
- **Intention:** Intention is the driving force of creation. Clearly define your intentions for the future, specifying what you want to manifest in your life. The clearer and more focused your intention, the more powerful your ability to co-create the future you desire.
- **Affirmations:** Affirmations are positive phrases that, when repeated with conviction, reprogram the subconscious and strengthen the belief in your ability to create the future you desire. Use affirmations that express your dreams and aspirations, repeating them daily with emotion and conviction.
- **Co-creation:** Co-creation is the process of creating in partnership with the universe, uniting your intention and action with the creative energy of the cosmos. The Arcturians teach us to trust the flow of life, following intuition and acting with confidence to manifest our dreams.
- **Release of Fears:** Fear is a powerful emotion that can paralyze us and prevent us from moving towards our dreams. Arcturian Future Healing helps us identify and release the fears that block us, opening space for confidence, courage, and action.

Applying Future Healing:
1. **Connection:** Connect with the Arcturian energy through meditation, conscious breathing, and invocation.
2. **Cleansing:** Free yourself from limiting expectations, fears, and negative beliefs that prevent you from dreaming big.
3. **Visualization:** Visualize the future you desire with clarity and emotion, feeling the experiences as if they were already happening.

4. **Intention:** Define your intentions for the future with clarity and focus, specifying what you want to manifest in your life.
5. **Affirmations:** Use positive affirmations to strengthen the belief in your ability to create the future you desire.
6. **Action:** Act with confidence and follow your intuition, co-creating the future in partnership with the universe.

Building a Radiant Future:

Arcturian Future Healing is an invitation to build the tomorrow you desire, free from fears, limitations, and uncertainties. By using the power of intention, visualization, and co-creation, you become the architect of your future, manifesting your dreams and aspirations with confidence and joy. Trust in the wisdom of the Arcturians, free yourself from the bonds of the past, and embrace the future with hope and enthusiasm. The future is yours to create!

Chapter 16
Healing the Physical Body

The physical body is a sacred temple that reflects the perfection and harmony of the vital energy that connects us to the universe. It is endowed with an innate intelligence that continuously seeks balance, even in the face of challenges imposed by routine and external factors. Arcturian Physical Body Healing is a process that awakens and enhances this innate capacity for regeneration and harmony, acting profoundly to restore vitality and promote integral well-being. By allowing universal energy to flow freely through each cell, the body becomes a fertile field for health, evidencing the synchronicity between matter and the energy that permeates it.

This healing method goes beyond simply mitigating physical symptoms. It acts on the energetic roots of health conditions, recognizing that imbalance in the physical body often originates in the subtle bodies. By addressing the underlying cause of disharmony, the Arcturian approach allows for complete restoration, where body, mind, and spirit align in a state of integration and fullness. Through practices such as energization, detoxification, and rejuvenation, the body is invited to return to its natural state of balance, reinforcing the connection with its vital essence.

Reconnecting with this bodily wisdom requires awareness and surrender. Listening attentively to the signals emitted by the body and practicing habits that respect its needs constitute the first steps to access this dimension of self-healing. When we nourish the body with quality foods, move it harmoniously, and cultivate positive thoughts, we initiate a cycle of regeneration and vitality. This care, aligned with Arcturian healing techniques, becomes a powerful tool to transform the body into a channel of pure energy, where health flourishes as an expression of the connection between the soul and the universe.

The Arcturians, with their deep knowledge of energy anatomy and human physiology, teach us that the physical body is a sacred vehicle, a temple that houses our soul and allows us to experience life on Earth. Arcturian Physical Body Healing is based on the principle that disease manifests first in the subtle bodies, later reflecting in the physical body. By treating the root cause of the disease at the energetic levels, Arcturian healing promotes physical, emotional, and spiritual well-being in an integrated and complete way.

Reconnecting with the Intelligence of the Body:

Your body has an innate wisdom, an intelligence that guides it in the search for balance and health. Arcturian Physical Body Healing helps you reconnect with this intelligence, awakening the power of self-healing and promoting well-being on all levels. By listening to your body's signals, nourishing it with healthy foods, moving it with joy, and cultivating positive thoughts and emotions, you will be honoring the sacred temple of your body and opening the way to health and vitality.

Arcturian Methods for Healing the Physical Body:

- **Energization:** The Arcturians use energization techniques to revitalize the physical body, increasing vitality, strengthening the immune system, and promoting cell regeneration. Through the channeling of vital energy, the laying on of hands, and the use of crystals, the Arcturians raise the vibratory frequency of the body, awakening the power of self-healing.
- **Detoxification:** The accumulation of toxins in the body can lead to various health problems. The Arcturians use energy detoxification techniques to remove toxins from the physical body and subtle bodies, promoting purification and rebalancing.
- **Rejuvenation:** Rejuvenation is a natural process that can be accelerated through Arcturian healing. The Arcturians

use techniques to activate collagen production, improve blood circulation, balance hormones, and promote cell regeneration, helping to maintain youthfulness and vitality.
- **Disease Healing:** Arcturian Physical Body Healing can be used to treat a wide range of diseases, from pain and inflammation to chronic and degenerative diseases. By treating the root cause of the disease at the energetic levels, Arcturian healing promotes physical healing and well-being in an integrated way.
- **Energy Surgery:** In more complex cases, the Arcturians can perform energy surgeries to remove blockages, repair tissues, and restore the flow of vital energy in the physical body. This non-invasive technique promotes healing quickly and effectively, without the need for physical interventions.

Applying Physical Body Healing:
1. **Intention:** Clearly define your intention for healing your physical body, specifying the areas you want to treat and the results you want to achieve.
2. **Connection:** Connect with Arcturian energy through meditation, conscious breathing, and invocation.
3. **Techniques:** Use Arcturian Physical Body Healing techniques that resonate with you, such as energization, detoxification, rejuvenation, and disease healing.
4. **Visualization:** Visualize Arcturian energy flowing through your body, healing every cell, organ, and system.
5. **Self-Care:** Cultivate healthy habits, such as a balanced diet, regular exercise, restful sleep, and contact with nature.
6. **Gratitude:** Thank your body for its wisdom and strength, recognizing it as a sacred temple that allows you to experience life on Earth.

Honoring the Sacred Temple of Your Body:
Arcturian Physical Body Healing is an invitation to honor the sacred temple of your body, reconnecting with its innate

intelligence and awakening the power of self-healing. By caring for your body with love, respect, and gratitude, you will be opening the way to health, vitality, and longevity. Trust the wisdom of the Arcturians, surrender to the healing process, and allow your body to become a channel of light, expressing the beauty and perfection of your soul.

Chapter 17
Emotional Healing

Emotions are an essential and transformative part of the human experience, acting as messengers that reveal our deepest needs and connect us with the flow of life. Arcturian Emotional Healing offers a path of liberation and balance, allowing repressed or misunderstood feelings to be embraced, processed, and transmuted into creative forces. This process promotes a state of serenity, self-knowledge, and inner harmony, unlocking limiting patterns and strengthening the power of love and joy in every aspect of existence.

Emotions are energies in motion that reflect our interaction with the internal and external world, but when not expressed adequately, they can accumulate as energetic charges that affect our physical, mental, and spiritual health. Arcturian Emotional Healing assists in the release of these charges, allowing feelings such as fear, sadness, and anger to be transformed into courage, gratitude, and trust. This process begins with the practice of acceptance and mindful observation, where each emotion is recognized as legitimate and valuable, opening the way to a deeper and more compassionate relationship with oneself.

Through specific practices such as conscious breathing, meditation, and emotional release techniques, Arcturian Emotional Healing promotes the purification and harmonization of the subtle bodies, creating a space for the true emotional essence to manifest. Creative expression is another pillar of this method, allowing art, writing, or movement to help externalize emotions, releasing blockages and opening space for new possibilities. This process culminates in a reconnection with joy and unconditional love, allowing you to reframe your experiences and strengthen your journey of evolution and emotional fullness.

The Arcturians, with their deep compassion and wisdom, understand the importance of emotions in our evolutionary journey. Emotions are energies in motion that connect us with life, drive us to act, and allow us to experience the richness of human experience. However, repressed emotions, unresolved traumas, and limiting emotional patterns can generate energy blockages, affecting our physical, mental, and spiritual health. Arcturian Emotional Healing guides us in releasing these blockages, transforming emotions into allies in our journey of growth and self-knowledge.

Understanding Your Emotions:

Each emotion you feel, be it joy, sadness, anger, or fear, carries an important message about your needs, your desires, and your challenges. Arcturian Emotional Healing invites you to embrace your emotions with compassion and curiosity, without judgment or resistance. By observing your emotions with mindfulness, you can understand their messages, identify their causes, and free yourself from the patterns that prevent you from living fully.

Arcturian Emotional Healing Techniques:

- **Identification:** The first step to emotional healing is to identify the emotions you are feeling. Pay attention to your body's signals, your thoughts, and behaviors. Name your emotions clearly and accurately, without judgment.
- **Acceptance:** Embrace your emotions with compassion and unconditional love, recognizing them as part of your human experience. Do not try to repress or deny your emotions, but rather welcome them as messengers that guide you on your journey.
- **Expression:** Express your emotions in a healthy and authentic way, whether through writing, art, dialogue, movement, or other forms of creative expression. Authentic expression of emotions releases blocked energy and promotes healing.

- **Release:** Use emotional release techniques, such as conscious breathing, meditation, and visualization, to release repressed emotions and traumas from the past. The Arcturians will guide you in this process, helping you to release dense energies and transform emotions into light.
- **Transmutation:** Transmutation is the process of transforming negative emotions into positive ones, using the energy of love and compassion. The Arcturians teach you to transmute anger into courage, fear into trust, and sadness into gratitude, raising your vibration and creating a more harmonious reality.
- **Inner Child Healing:** Arcturian Emotional Healing also focuses on healing the inner child, that part of us that carries the wounds and traumas of childhood. By healing the inner child, you free yourself from patterns of abandonment, rejection, and insecurity, reconnecting with joy, spontaneity, and unconditional love.

Applying Emotional Healing:

1. **Self-Observation:** Cultivate self-observation, paying attention to your thoughts, emotions, and behaviors.
2. **Emotional Journal:** Keep an emotional journal to record your emotions, identify your triggers, and track your progress in emotional healing.
3. **Release Techniques:** Use emotional release techniques, such as conscious breathing, meditation, and visualization, to release repressed emotions.
4. **Creative Expression:** Express your emotions through art, music, writing, or other forms of creative expression.
5. **Self-Care:** Prioritize self-care, taking care of your body, mind, and spirit through practices that bring you well-being.
6. **Compassion:** Cultivate compassion for yourself and others, recognizing that we are all on a journey of learning and healing.

Freeing Yourself to Love and Be Happy:

Arcturian Emotional Healing is an invitation to free yourself from the patterns that prevent you from loving and being happy. By embracing, transforming, and releasing your emotions, you open space for inner peace, balance, and fullness. Trust the wisdom of the Arcturians, surrender to the healing process, and allow your emotions to guide you towards your true essence.

Chapter 18
Mental Healing

The mind is an unlimited space of creation and transformation, where each thought has the power to shape the reality we experience. With the practice of Arcturian Mental Healing, it is possible to transcend the barriers of limiting beliefs and negative thought patterns, accessing a state of clarity and mental serenity. This process promotes alignment between the higher consciousness and the inner world, allowing the mind to become a channel of conscious manifestation, full of peace and creativity. From this reconnection, the ability to create a reality more aligned with your dreams and purpose emerges.

The thoughts we cultivate are seeds sown in our mental field, and it is up to each of us to decide which ones to nurture. Positive thoughts aligned with constructive intentions flourish in experiences of fulfillment and harmony, while those rooted in fear or doubt generate obstacles. The practice of Arcturian Mental Healing teaches us to observe the mind with mindfulness, recognizing patterns that no longer serve growth and reprogramming them with empowering beliefs. This transformation is the key to freeing oneself from cycles of anxiety and self-sabotage, opening space for the flourishing of ideas and achievements.

With the use of tools such as meditation, visualization, and belief reprogramming, the mind is trained to align with the highest vibrations, allowing inner wisdom and mental focus to integrate into everyday life. The constant practice of these techniques not only promotes calm and balance but also expands the ability to access insights and creative solutions to life's challenges. Thus, the mind ceases to be a space of restlessness and becomes a temple of serenity and manifestation, where peace and power coexist harmoniously.

The Arcturians, with their advanced understanding of the human mind, teach us that our thoughts are like seeds that we plant in our mental garden. Positive and constructive thoughts generate fruits of happiness, abundance, and fulfillment, while negative and limiting thoughts create weeds that suffocate our potential and prevent us from flourishing. Arcturian Mental Healing empowers us to cultivate a fertile and abundant mental garden where inner peace, clarity, and creativity flourish in harmony.

Mastering Your Thoughts:

The human mind is a powerful tool, capable of creating wonderful realities or trapping us in cycles of suffering. Arcturian Mental Healing invites us to take control of our thoughts, becoming aware of the mental patterns that limit us and cultivating positive and constructive thoughts that propel us towards our dreams.

Arcturian Mental Healing Techniques:
- **Observation:** The first step to mental healing is to observe your thoughts without judgment. Pay attention to your inner dialogues, identify repeating thought patterns, and recognize the limiting beliefs that prevent you from reaching your full potential.
- **Reprogramming:** Once you have identified the limiting beliefs, it is time to reprogram them. Use positive affirmations, visualizations, and NLP (Neuro-Linguistic Programming) techniques to replace negative beliefs with beliefs that empower you and propel you towards your goals.
- **Meditation:** Meditation is a powerful tool to calm the mind, reduce stress, and cultivate inner peace. Through meditation, you can connect with your inner wisdom, receive insights, and access higher states of consciousness.
- **Visualization:** Visualization is a technique that uses the power of imagination to create the reality you desire.

Visualize yourself achieving your goals, living with health, abundance, and happiness. Visualization sends a clear signal to the universe, attracting into your life the people, situations, and opportunities that resonate with your dreams.
- **Energy Healing:** The Arcturians use energy healing techniques to harmonize your chakras, balance your subtle bodies, and dissolve negative energy patterns that may be affecting your mental and emotional health.

Applying Mental Healing:

1. **Mindfulness:** Cultivate mindfulness, observing your thoughts without judgment.
2. **Thought Journal:** Keep a thought journal to record your mental patterns, identify limiting beliefs, and track your progress in mental healing.
3. **Affirmations:** Use positive affirmations to reprogram limiting beliefs and strengthen constructive thoughts.
4. **Meditation:** Practice meditation regularly to calm the mind, reduce stress, and cultivate inner peace.
5. **Visualization:** Use visualization to create the reality you desire, imagining yourself achieving your goals and living with fullness.
6. **Gratitude:** Cultivate gratitude for your positive thoughts and the opportunities that life offers you.

Cultivating a serene and powerful mind is an act of profound self-care and self-mastery. By integrating Arcturian Mental Healing practices into your routine, you access a state of inner balance that directly reflects in the quality of your life and your achievements. Each realigned thought, each transformed belief, is a step towards a more conscious and harmonious existence. In this process, the mind becomes fertile ground where dreams and intentions flourish, connecting you with the infinite potential of the universe and allowing peace and clarity to be the foundation of your journey.

Chapter 19
Spiritual Healing

Spirituality is the essence that connects every being to the infinite, revealing the divine presence that permeates all things. Through Arcturian Spiritual Healing, this sacred bond is intensified, leading to the expansion of consciousness and the awakening of the true inner nature. This process transcends the limitations imposed by the ego, dissolves energy blocks, and expands the perception of oneness with the Divine. With practices that raise the vibration and align the physical, mental and energy bodies, it becomes possible to access a dimension of peace, wisdom and unconditional love, fundamental for the evolution of the soul and for the fulfillment of the greater purpose.

The spiritual journey begins with the recognition that the divine essence dwells within each being. This awareness allows us to overcome the illusions that generate fear, doubt and separation, guiding us to a life more aligned with the values of compassion and self-knowledge. Arcturian Spiritual Healing assists in this awakening through practices that harmonize the chakras, strengthen the connection with the Higher Self and promote a deep energetic purification. Thus, the individual frees himself from limiting patterns, opening himself to a more expansive life experience, in tune with the higher realms and with the wisdom of the universe.

By integrating techniques such as meditation, working with spirit guides and activating the Merkaba, Spiritual Healing transforms the body into a vehicle of light capable of accessing higher dimensions. These practices not only promote inner peace, but also create a deep alignment with the soul's mission, helping to manifest the unique talents and gifts of each being. This journey of ascension is not only individual, but also a contribution to the collective elevation of planetary consciousness, an essential step in building a more harmonious and enlightened future.

The Arcturians, beings of light who vibrate in higher dimensions, understand spirituality as the essence of life, the force that connects us with the divine source and propels us towards evolution. Arcturian Spiritual Healing invites us to transcend the limitations of the ego, awaken to our true nature and manifest our divine potential. It is a journey of self-knowledge, healing and expansion of consciousness that leads us to union with the Divine and the fulfillment of our soul purpose.

Awakening Consciousness:

The awakening of consciousness is a gradual process that begins with the recognition of our true divine nature. It is a call to transcend the illusions of the ego, free ourselves from limiting beliefs and connect with the wisdom, love and peace that reside within us. Arcturian Spiritual Healing assists us in this process, raising our vibration, purifying our subtle bodies and opening our hearts to the experience of the Divine.

Arcturian Spiritual Healing Techniques:

- **Meditation:** Meditation is a fundamental practice for the awakening of consciousness and connection with the Higher Self. Through meditation, you can calm the mind, silence the ego and access higher states of consciousness, where intuition, wisdom and connection with the Divine manifest clearly.
- **Connection with the Higher Self:** The Higher Self is your divine essence, your divine spark that resides in higher dimensions. Through Arcturian Spiritual Healing, you can strengthen your connection with the Higher Self, receiving guidance, healing and inspiration for your journey.
- **Chakra Healing:** Chakras are energy centers that connect the physical body to the subtle bodies. Arcturian Spiritual Healing uses techniques to harmonize and balance the

chakras, promoting the free flow of vital energy and the awakening of consciousness.
- **Working with Spirit Guides:** Spirit guides are beings of light who accompany us on our evolutionary journey, offering guidance, protection and support. Arcturian Spiritual Healing teaches us to connect with our spirit guides, receiving their messages and learning from their wisdom.
- **Merkaba Activation:** The Merkaba is the vehicle of light that transports us to higher dimensions. Arcturian Spiritual Healing uses techniques to activate the Merkaba, facilitating astral travel, spiritual ascension and connection with the higher realms.

Applying Spiritual Healing:
1. **Spiritual Practice:** Cultivate a daily spiritual practice, such as meditation, prayer, study of sacred texts or connection with nature.
2. **Intention:** Set the intention to connect with your divine essence and walk the path of ascension.
3. **Meditation:** Meditate regularly to calm the mind, silence the ego and access higher states of consciousness.
4. **Invocation:** Invoke the presence of the Arcturians and your spirit guides, requesting guidance and assistance on your spiritual journey.
5. **Self-knowledge:** Dedicate yourself to self-knowledge, exploring your beliefs, values and life purpose.
6. **Service:** Put your gifts and talents at the service of others, contributing to the elevation of planetary consciousness.

Spiritual Healing is an invitation to reintegrate with the divine essence that dwells in each being, a journey of rediscovery that transcends limits and aligns us with the greater purpose of existence. As we delve deeper into the practices and allow ourselves to be guided by Arcturian wisdom, life takes on a new perspective, full of meaning, clarity and connection with the Whole. On this path, we not only awaken to our spiritual nature, but also become catalysts for transformation and light for the world, manifesting a more harmonious reality in tune with the universal principles of love and unity.

Chapter 20
Soul Healing

The soul, the center of our divine essence, holds the totality of our experiences, both those that have uplifted us and those that have challenged us. Its eternal nature reflects a journey of continuous learning and growth, marked by cycles of light and shadow. Arcturian Soul Healing offers a profound and transformative path to release wounds, traumas and karmic patterns that can obscure its light and limit its potential. This process promotes a loving reconnection with your most authentic self, awakening the ability to live fully, aligned with the wisdom and unconditional love that permeate the universe.

Soul wounds, often rooted in experiences from this or other lifetimes, can manifest as persistent fears, feelings of inadequacy, patterns of self-sabotage, or difficulty connecting deeply with love and joy. Recognizing these wounds is the first step on the healing journey. With the compassionate support of the Arcturians, it is possible to access significant memories, understand the origins of blockages and transform them into enriching learning. On this path, practices such as regression, forgiveness and shadow integration act as powerful tools to release dense energy and restore inner harmony.

By embracing the totality of your being - light and shadow - you open yourself to the experience of unconditional love, the primordial force that heals, transforms and unites. This love, when directed to yourself and to all beings, dissolves the barriers of the ego, allowing you to perceive yourself as an inseparable part of a greater whole. Arcturian Soul Healing invites the intentional practice of forgiveness, the loving acceptance of all facets of your existence and the conscious manifestation of your divine essence. With this, the soul finds its fullness, radiating light, wisdom and peace in every aspect of its journey.

The soul, the divine spark that resides within us, carries the history of our experiences, our joys, our pains and our learnings throughout countless lifetimes. Deep emotional wounds, unresolved traumas and karmic patterns can create blockages in the soul, preventing us from manifesting our true essence and living fully. Arcturian Soul Healing invites us to dive into the depths of our being, recognizing and healing the wounds of the soul, freeing ourselves from limiting patterns and awakening to the light, love and wisdom that reside within us.

Recognizing Soul Wounds:

Soul wounds manifest in a variety of ways, such as patterns of self-sabotage, difficulty connecting with love, fear of rejection, feelings of guilt and shame, among others. Arcturian Soul Healing helps us to recognize these wounds, understand their origins and release the blocked energies that prevent us from living fully.

Arcturian Soul Healing Techniques:

- **Regression:** Regression, guided by the Arcturians, allows you to access memories of past lives, identifying the origin of karmic patterns, traumas and blockages that manifest in your present life. By understanding the root of these patterns, you can release blocked energies and begin the process of soul healing.
- **Forgiveness:** Forgiveness is a balm for the soul, freeing us from the weight of the past and opening space for healing and love. Forgiving yourself and others for past hurts and resentments, whether from this life or past lives, allows the soul to free itself from the bonds of resentment and guilt, finding inner peace and freedom.
- **Shadow Integration:** The shadow is the part of us that we reject, that we hide from ourselves and others. It contains our fears, our insecurities, our anger and all the emotions and qualities that we consider negative or unacceptable. Arcturian Soul Healing invites us to integrate the shadow,

recognizing it as part of ourselves and welcoming it with love and compassion. By integrating the shadow, we recover the totality of our being, accessing the strength, creativity and wisdom that were hidden within us.
- **Awakening Unconditional Love:** Unconditional love is the most powerful force in the universe, capable of healing all wounds and connecting us with our divine essence. Arcturian Soul Healing helps us to awaken unconditional love for ourselves and for all beings, transcending the barriers of the ego and opening our hearts to the experience of unity.

Applying Soul Healing:
1. **Intention:** Set the intention to heal your soul, freeing yourself from karmic patterns and awakening to the fullness of your being.
2. **Connection:** Connect with the Arcturian energy through meditation, conscious breathing and invocation.
3. **Self-knowledge:** Dedicate yourself to self-knowledge, exploring your emotions, your thoughts and your behaviors.
4. **Forgiveness:** Practice forgiveness, freeing yourself from the weight of the past and opening space for healing and love.
5. **Shadow Integration:** Recognize and embrace your shadow, integrating it with love and compassion.
6. **Unconditional Love:** Cultivate unconditional love for yourself and for all beings, opening your heart to the experience of unity.

Arcturian Soul Healing is an invitation to awaken to the fullness of your being, reconnecting with your divine essence, freeing yourself from karmic patterns and opening your heart to unconditional love. By healing your soul, you will be walking the path of ascension, manifesting your true essence and co-creating a future of light, harmony and abundance. Trust in the wisdom of the Arcturians, surrender to the healing process and allow your soul to expand, radiant and free, towards the light.

Chapter 21
Healing the Planet

Human consciousness has the power to transcend the limitations of individualism and embrace a deeper connection with the planet, recognizing it as a living being, conscious and interconnected with all its inhabitants. Planetary healing is not just a responsibility, but a call for collective transformation, where every action, thought and intention resonates in the network of energies that sustains the Earth. Through Arcturian wisdom, we are invited to access a higher state of consciousness that allows us to perceive Gaia as a living, pulsating and compassionate force that nourishes and sustains us. With this perception, comes the opportunity to harmonize telluric energies, restore natural cycles and contribute to a balanced and sustainable future.

By integrating energy healing practices, targeted meditations and a deep connection with the elementals of nature, we awaken our ability to act as catalysts for planetary regeneration. Through these practices, we can visualize Arcturian energies flowing through the planet, purifying wounded areas and revitalizing the vital network that connects all beings. We recognize that every act of gratitude, care and respect for nature has a tangible impact on Gaia's health, resonating in all dimensions of existence. Thus, healing the planet is not just a solution to ecological challenges, but a path to collective elevation, where love, compassion and responsibility converge to create a reality of peace and harmony.

Understanding Earth as an interconnected system inspires us to take conscious action in our daily lives, promoting sustainable practices and honoring life in all its forms. Whether through reducing consumption, conscious use of natural resources or education about the importance of environmental preservation, every gesture contributes to the restoration of ecological balance. The loving energy of Gaia and the support of the Arcturians remind us that by healing the planet, we also heal ourselves, for we are intrinsically connected to the Earth in body, mind and spirit. This is a journey of co-creation, where the vision of a radiant and harmonious future becomes a manifested reality through the union of efforts and awakened consciousness.

The Arcturians, with their holistic and compassionate vision, understand Earth as a living being, conscious and interconnected with all the beings that inhabit it. Gaia, the soul of the planet, is a powerful force that nourishes, sustains and guides us on our evolutionary journey. However, pollution, the unbridled exploitation of natural resources and disharmony in the collective consciousness have caused deep wounds in Gaia, affecting the ecological balance and the health of the planet. Arcturian Planet Healing invites us to awaken to our responsibility as guardians of the Earth, uniting our hearts and minds to heal the wounds of the past, restore balance and co-create a sustainable and harmonious future for all beings.

Connecting with Gaia Consciousness:

Gaia Consciousness is the soul of the planet, a living and intelligent force that permeates all beings and ecosystems on Earth. By connecting with Gaia, we awaken to the interconnection of all life forms, recognizing that we are part of a greater whole and that our actions directly impact the health of the planet. Arcturian Planet Healing teaches us to tune into Gaia's vibration, listening to her messages, honoring her wisdom and contributing to her healing and well-being.

Arcturian Planet Healing Techniques:

- **Planetary Meditation:** Planetary meditation is a powerful practice to connect with Gaia Consciousness, send light and healing to the planet and co-create a harmonious future for all beings. Visualize the Earth enveloped in a mantle of light, imagine lush forests, crystal clear oceans

and all living beings vibrating in harmony. Send love and gratitude to Gaia, recognizing her wisdom and strength.
- **Earth Energy Healing:** The Arcturians use energy healing techniques to harmonize telluric energies, purify the planet's energy points and restore balance to ecosystems. Visualize Arcturian energy flowing through the Earth, healing the wounds of the past, removing energy blockages and revitalizing the planet.
- **Alignment with Elementals:** Elementals are the spirits of nature that inhabit earth, water, fire and air. They are guardians of nature and can assist in healing the planet. Connect with the elementals, honoring their wisdom and requesting their collaboration in healing the Earth.
- **Co-creating a Sustainable Future:** Arcturian Planet Healing invites us to co-create a sustainable future where humanity lives in harmony with nature, respecting all living beings and using natural resources consciously and responsibly. Visualize a future where abundance, peace and harmony prevail, and act in your daily life to manifest this reality.

Applying Planet Healing:
1. **Connection:** Connect with Gaia Consciousness through meditation, contact with nature and expressing gratitude for life.
2. **Energy Healing:** Send light and healing to the planet through visualization, planetary meditation and the use of crystals.
3. **Sustainable Actions:** Adopt sustainable practices in your daily life, such as reducing consumption, reusing materials, recycling, planting trees and consuming organic and locally produced products.
4. **Respect for Nature:** Cultivate respect for all living beings, preserving nature and protecting animals.
5. **Collective Consciousness:** Share your knowledge about planet healing, inspiring others to join this mission of love and healing.

Arcturian Planet Healing is a call to awaken as guardians of the Earth, uniting our hearts and minds to heal the wounds of the past, restore balance and co-create a sustainable and harmonious future for all beings. Trust in the wisdom of the Arcturians, surrender to the flow of life and allow the loving energy of Gaia to guide you on your journey of healing and ascension. Together, we can create a radiant future for our planet and for all life forms that inhabit it.

Chapter 22
Distance Healing

Distance healing transcends the barriers of space and time, allowing loving and healing energy to reach any person, animal, or situation, regardless of their physical location. This process is a direct expression of the principle of universal interconnection, in which all beings are linked by an invisible network of energy. Through clear intention, focused visualization, and connection with higher planes, it is possible to channel transformative energies that promote balance, harmonization, and restoration. This practice, amplified by Arcturian wisdom, offers us a powerful means of exerting a positive impact on both individual and collective levels, bringing relief and well-being to those who need it most.

The Arcturians, with their deep multidimensional understanding, teach that distance healing is sustained by the force of pure intention, which acts as a catalyst to direct energy with precision and effectiveness. Through this technique, we are able to create an energetic link with whomever we wish to help, channeling light and love that adjust to the specific needs of each being or situation. This connection does not depend on physical or temporal limitations, but is established through the resonance of our vibrations with the universal energy network. Thus, by practicing distance healing, we become conscious channels of transformation, amplifying the possibilities of well-being and balance.

To apply distance healing ethically and effectively, it is essential to respect free will and the unique process of each being. Before sending energy, connect with your own inner source of light, invoking the loving presence of the Arcturians to guide and amplify your intentions. Visualize the person, animal, or situation enveloped in radiant light, imagining the energy flowing smoothly and promoting healing and harmony. Whether to help someone in suffering, restore balance to a place, or contribute to planetary regeneration, each act of healing is also an act of unconditional love. Through this practice, we expand our capacity to serve and participate in building a more harmonious world full of light.

The Arcturians, with their advanced technology and understanding of multidimensional energy, have mastered the art of distance healing. They teach us that energy is not limited to physical space, but can be sent and directed through intention, visualization, and connection with higher planes. Arcturian Distance Healing empowers us to transcend physical limitations, becoming channels of healing and love for those in need, whether they are near or far.

Principles of Distance Healing:
- **Interconnection:** Distance Healing is based on the principle of interconnection of all beings and all things. We are all connected by an invisible energetic web, and the energy we send to another reverberates throughout the universe.
- **Intention:** Intention is the driving force of distance healing. Clearly define your intention to send healing, love, and harmonization to the person, animal, or situation you wish to help.
- **Visualization:** Visualization is a powerful tool for directing healing energy. Imagine the person or situation you wish to heal, surrounding them with light and sending loving energy.
- **Connection with the Arcturians:** Invoke the presence of the Arcturians, requesting their assistance and guidance in distance healing. Visualize Arcturian energy flowing through you, amplifying the power of healing.

Distance Healing Techniques:

- **Sending Energy:** Sit or lie down comfortably, close your eyes, and connect with Arcturian energy. Visualize the person or situation you wish to heal, surrounding them with light and sending loving energy through your hands or your heart chakra.
- **Distance Treatment:** Perform a complete distance treatment using the Arcturian healing techniques you have already learned, such as etheric laying on of hands, energy surgery, chromotherapy, and crystal healing. Visualize the person receiving the treatment, feeling the benefits of healing.
- **Planetary Healing:** Send healing energy to planet Earth, visualizing Gaia enveloped in light, harmonizing telluric energies and promoting ecological balance.
- **Healing of Humanity:** Send healing energy to humanity, visualizing all human beings connected in love, peace, and harmony.

Ethics of Distance Healing:

- **Permission:** Before sending distance healing to someone, ask permission from the person or their Higher Self. Respect everyone's free will.
- **Pure Intention:** Send healing with pure intention, without attachment to the outcome. Trust in the wisdom of the universe and the self-healing capacity of each being.
- **Responsibility:** Recognize that you are a channel of healing, but true healing comes from within each being. Do not take responsibility for another's healing process.

Applying Distance Healing:

1. **Preparation:** Prepare for distance healing by creating a sacred space, connecting with your heart, and invoking the presence of the Arcturians.
2. **Intention:** Clearly define your intention for distance healing, specifying the person, animal, or situation you wish to help.

3. **Visualization:** Visualize the person or situation you wish to heal, surrounding them with light and sending loving energy.
4. **Techniques:** Use Arcturian Distance Healing techniques that resonate with you, such as sending energy, distance treatment, and planetary healing.
5. **Gratitude:** Thank the Arcturians for their assistance and the universe for the opportunity to be a channel of healing and love.

Arcturian Distance Healing expands the reach of healing, allowing you to contribute to the well-being of people, animals, and the planet as a whole. By mastering this technique, you become an agent of healing and transformation, bringing light and love to all corners of the universe. Trust in the wisdom of the Arcturians, surrender to the flow of healing energy, and allow unconditional love to guide your actions.

Chapter 23
Arcturian Technology

The secrets of Arcturian Technology reveal a dimension of healing and evolution that integrates advanced science and spiritual principles in perfect harmony. Through extraordinary devices and revolutionary methods, the Arcturians offer a glimpse into a future where well-being is addressed in an integral way, contemplating body, mind, and spirit. The essence of this technology lies in the precise manipulation of vibrational energies, lights and sounds, capable of rebalancing the human being at deep levels. More than mere tools, these resources are extensions of the Arcturians' higher consciousness, used to assist humanity on its journey of ascension and expansion of consciousness.

The healing chambers exemplify this transformative power. Designed with technology that transcends the known laws of physics, these structures emanate vibrations that act directly on cells, tissues and energy bodies, promoting regeneration and well-being at all levels. These sophisticated devices go beyond the physical aspect, helping to dissolve emotional traumas and unlock spiritual potentials. In addition, etheric crystals are another vital component of this technology, operating as multidimensional energy sources. They amplify the individual's vibration, restoring the balance of the chakras and activating dormant light codes in DNA, which contributes to a state of harmony and fullness.

Connection with higher dimensions is also a central aspect of Arcturian Technology. Through dimensional portals, these advanced beings can access different realities and share their wisdom with other civilizations. These portals not only facilitate movement between worlds, but also expand human perception, allowing a more intimate contact with higher levels of existence. The use of energy probes for diagnosis and healing demonstrates the precision of these practices, identifying blockages and promoting fine-tuning in the subtle bodies. Each innovation reflects an ethical and compassionate approach, reinforcing the Arcturian commitment to the preservation and advancement of life in its highest form.

Arcturian Technology is not just a demonstration of technical progress; it represents a model of how science and spirituality can coexist to transform lives. The wisdom of these interdimensional masters is not limited by duality or the constraints of human thought. Instead, it invites us to rethink our vision of health, evolution, and purpose, offering tools to co-create a future where love and consciousness guide humanity towards fulfillment.

The Arcturians, with their advanced civilization and deep knowledge of the universe, master technologies that seem like science fiction to our eyes. But for them, technology is an extension of consciousness, a tool to manifest love, healing, and evolution. Arcturian Technology is based on the manipulation of energy, vibration and consciousness, using frequencies, crystals, light and sound to promote harmonization, balance and ascension.

HEALING CHAMBERS:

Arcturian healing chambers are advanced devices that use light, sound and vibrational frequencies to promote physical, emotional and spiritual healing. Imagine yourself entering a healing chamber, surrounded by multicolored lights, harmonious sounds and subtle vibrations that penetrate every cell of your being, removing blockages, regenerating tissues and raising your vibration. Arcturian healing chambers can assist in the treatment of diseases, rejuvenation, DNA activation and expansion of consciousness.

ETHERIC CRYSTALS:

Etheric crystals are forms of crystalline energy that vibrate in higher dimensions, emitting frequencies that promote healing and ascension. The Arcturians use etheric crystals in their healing technologies, amplifying energy, harmonizing the chakras and activating light codes in DNA. Imagine an etheric crystal being projected into your body, dissolving energy blockages, balancing your subtle bodies and raising your vibration.

ENERGY PROBES:

Energy probes are instruments used by Arcturians to perform accurate energy diagnoses and treatments. Imagine an energy probe traversing your energy field, identifying blockages, imbalances and disease patterns. Energy probes can be used to remove negative energies, repair damage to subtle bodies and promote healing at deep levels.

DIMENSIONAL PORTALS:

Dimensional portals are openings in the fabric of space-time that allow travel between different dimensions. The Arcturians use dimensional portals to access Earth and other planets, bringing their wisdom and technology to assist in the evolution of humanity. Imagine going through a dimensional portal, accessing higher realities and expanding your consciousness beyond the limits of the third dimension.

Other Arcturian technologies:
- Starships: Arcturian starships are advanced vehicles that use energy to move through space, transcending the laws of physics as we know them. They are capable of traveling through dimensional portals, accessing different realities and carrying out healing and planetary assistance missions.
- Arcturian Robots: The Arcturians use advanced robots to assist in their tasks, performing work that requires precision, strength or endurance. These robots are programmed with artificial intelligence and compassion, acting in harmony with human beings and nature.
- Communication technology: The Arcturians communicate through telepathy, channeling and advanced technologies that allow the transmission of information instantly, regardless of distance.

The Ethics of Arcturian Technology:

Arcturian Technology is used with wisdom, compassion and respect for life. The Arcturians are concerned with ethics and safety in all their actions, ensuring that technology is used for the good of humanity and the planet.

Arcturian Technology offers us a glimpse into the future of healing, where science and spirituality come together to promote well-being, evolution and ascension. By opening ourselves to this new era of healing, we are expanding our consciousness, awakening our divine potential and co-creating a radiant future for humanity.

Chapter 24
Quantum Leap

The Quantum Leap represents a profound and expansive transformation of human consciousness, allowing the transcendence of three-dimensional limitations and direct connection with the multidimensional nature of being. It is a dynamic and accelerated process in which individual energetic vibration is raised to higher frequencies, unlocking new perceptions, abilities and realities. In this elevated state, the rigid boundaries of human experience dissolve, revealing an interconnected universe where the unlimited potential of each individual can be manifested. This transformation is not merely a single event, but a continuous invitation to live in alignment with higher dimensions of existence and access a broader understanding of reality.

The role of the Arcturians in this process is fundamental, as they act as compassionate guides and masters of ascension. The energy emitted by these high vibrational beings facilitates the gradual adjustment of human frequency, allowing the transition to occur safely and harmoniously. Through advanced technologies and methods such as DNA activation, the Arcturians awaken light codes that reside dormant in the genetic core, expanding perception and preparing the individual for a higher level of consciousness. In addition, their energy healing practices act on the release of blockages and harmonization of the subtle bodies, creating an energy field conducive to vibrational leap.

This awakening is not only technical or energetic, but also deeply transformative on an emotional and mental level. During the Quantum Leap, it becomes crucial to release old beliefs, traumas and limiting patterns that restrict the experience of who we truly are. The connection with Arcturian energy offers continuous support to face the challenges of this purification, helping to cultivate inner peace and balance. This journey transforms not only the way we perceive the world, but also how we position ourselves within it, allowing us to operate from a higher perspective, guided by love, compassion and understanding of unity.

Living the Quantum Leap means embarking on a journey of continuous self-discovery and expansion, allowing each experience and each insight to strengthen your connection with the higher self and with the universal flow of life. It not only expands individual consciousness, but also contributes to the collective awakening of humanity, creating a world where light, harmony and unity prevail. Trusting the process, aligning with higher energies and remaining open to transformations are essential steps to fully integrate this new reality and co-create a higher and more meaningful existence.

The Quantum Leap is an evolutionary leap, a vibrational shift that elevates your consciousness to a new level of perception and understanding of reality. It is as if you are tuning your frequency to a higher radio station, accessing information, energies and realities that were previously beyond your reach. The Arcturians, with their deep wisdom and experience in ascension, guide us in this process, helping us to release the bonds that bind us to the third dimension and awaken to our true multidimensional nature.

The Nature of Reality:

Reality, as we perceive it, is a construct of our consciousness. Our thoughts, beliefs and emotions shape our experience, creating the illusion of a solid and separate world. The Quantum Leap invites us to question this perception, opening ourselves to the possibility that reality is much more fluid and interconnected than we imagine. By transcending the limitations of the third dimension, we awaken to our true multidimensional nature, connecting with infinite possibilities and realities.

How Arcturian Energy Assists in the Quantum Leap:

The Arcturians, with their advanced technology and knowledge of consciousness, use various tools to assist in the Quantum Leap:

- Raising Vibration: The Arcturians emit high vibrational frequencies that assist in raising your frequency, facilitating the transition to higher dimensions.
- DNA Activation: DNA activation, as we saw in chapter 12, awakens dormant light codes, expanding your consciousness and paving the way for new abilities and perceptions.
- Energy Healing: Arcturian energy healing removes blockages, harmonizes the chakras and balances the subtle bodies, preparing you for the expansion of consciousness.
- Expansion of Consciousness: The Arcturians use techniques to expand your consciousness, helping you to transcend the limitations of the ego and connect with your divine essence.
- Guidance and Support: The Arcturians offer guidance and support during the Quantum Leap process, helping you navigate the changes and challenges that arise during ascension.

Preparing for the Quantum Leap:

- Raise your Vibration: Cultivate positive thoughts and emotions, practice meditation, connect with nature and use other techniques to raise your vibration.
- Release the Past: Free yourself from traumas, limiting beliefs and patterns from the past that prevent you from moving forward on your evolutionary journey.
- Heal Your Emotions: Embrace and transform your emotions, cultivating inner peace and emotional balance.
- Expand Your Mind: Question your beliefs, seek new knowledge and open yourself to new perspectives and realities.

- Connect with your Higher Self: Strengthen your connection with your Higher Self, seeking guidance and inspiration for your journey.

Living the Quantum Leap:

The Quantum Leap is a gradual process that manifests in different ways for each person. You may experience changes in your perception of reality, increased intuition, synchronicities, vivid dreams, access to new information and skills, among other experiences. Trust the process, stay open to change and allow Arcturian energy to guide you on your journey of ascension.

The Quantum Leap is an invitation to transcend the limitations of the third dimension and awaken to your true multidimensional nature. It is a journey of expansion of consciousness, of connection with your unlimited potential and of co-creation of a new reality. Trust in the wisdom of the Arcturians, surrender to the flow of life and allow the Quantum Leap to propel you to a new level of consciousness, where light, love and harmony prevail.

Chapter 25
Astral Travel

Astral Travel is an extraordinary experience that transcends the limits of the physical body and offers the opportunity to explore the vastness of the universe and higher dimensions. This process allows the conscious projection of your essence in a state of complete freedom, where consciousness moves through the astral plane, accessing hidden knowledge, interacting with spiritual guides, and experiencing realities beyond the tangible. This practice, widely recognized for its ability to expand perception and accelerate spiritual growth, invites us to experience reality in a broader way, revealing our multidimensional nature and the infinite potential of the human being.

Guided by ancestral techniques and the advanced wisdom of the Arcturians, Astral Travel is an invitation to break internal and external barriers, starting with a deep state of relaxation. In this state, the physical body is left at rest while the astral body, an energetic extension of your consciousness, emerges to explore subtle dimensions. Careful visualizations and intentional affirmations help to direct this experience, allowing the astral traveler to choose specific destinations and purposes for the journey, whether to seek self-knowledge, visit energetic places, or interact with beings of light.

An essential element of Astral Travel is the silver cord, an energetic link that maintains a secure connection between the physical body and the astral body throughout the experience. This link provides security to the traveler, ensuring that they can return to the physical body at any time with ease and integrity. The guidance of the Arcturians plays an important role in this process, offering energetic protection and guidance so that the exploration of the astral plane is done consciously and responsibly. Practices such as creating a protective light field around the astral body, establishing clear intentions, and actively seeking guidance from spiritual guides are essential for a safe and enriching experience.

After the experience, integrating the lessons learned on the astral plane is as important as the journey itself. Conscious reflections, journaling, and meditation practices help to understand the insights received, allowing this knowledge to become part of everyday life. Astral Travel, when conducted with respect and responsibility, not only broadens spiritual horizons but also strengthens the individual's connection with the universe, promoting a state of harmony, self-discovery, and continuous growth.

Astral Travel, also known as consciousness projection, is an experience in which you separate from your physical body and travel with your astral body to other dimensions of reality. It is an opportunity to explore the universe, access hidden knowledge, connect with spiritual guides, and experience freedom and the expansion of consciousness. The Arcturians, masters in the art of interdimensional travel, guide us in this process, sharing their wisdom and techniques so we can explore the astral plane with safety and awareness.

Understanding Astral Travel:

During Astral Travel, your consciousness separates from the physical body and projects itself onto the astral plane, a subtle dimension of reality that interpenetrates the physical world. In this state, you can travel anywhere in the universe, visit different dimensions, encounter beings of light, and access information that is beyond the reach of the conscious mind. Astral Travel is a transformative experience that expands consciousness, accelerates spiritual growth, and connects you with the vastness of the universe.

Techniques for Astral Projection:

- **Relaxation:** Relax your body and mind through breathing techniques, meditation, or progressive muscle relaxation.

Deep relaxation is essential for consciousness to detach from the physical body.
- **Visualization:** Visualize yourself floating out of your body, observing it from above. Imagine yourself traveling to the place you want to visit, be it a physical place, a higher dimension, or an encounter with a spiritual guide.
- **Affirmations:** Use affirmations that express your intention to perform Astral Travel safely and consciously. Mentally repeat phrases like "I project myself on the astral plane with safety and awareness" or "I am in control of my astral experience."
- **Energy Techniques:** Use energy techniques to strengthen your astral body and facilitate projection. Visualize your astral body vibrant and luminous, enveloped in protective light.
- **Silver Cord:** During Astral Travel, you remain connected to your physical body through a silver cord, an energetic thread that ensures your safe return. Visualize the silver cord connecting your astral body to your physical body, ensuring your safety during the journey.

Exploring the Astral Plane Safely:
- **Protection:** Before starting Astral Travel, invoke the protection of the Arcturians, angels, or spiritual guides. Visualize yourself surrounded by white light, creating a protective shield around you.
- **Intention:** Clearly define your intention for Astral Travel. Where do you want to go? What do you want to learn or experience?
- **Control:** Remember that you are in control of your astral experience. If you feel fear or discomfort, affirm your intention to return to your physical body.
- **Spiritual Guides:** Connect with your spiritual guides during Astral Travel, requesting their guidance and protection.
- **Return:** When you want to return to your physical body, visualize yourself floating back and reconnecting to your

body. Move your fingers and toes to reconnect with physical reality.

Integrating Learnings:

After the astral journey, take some time to integrate the learnings and insights you have received. Write down your experiences in a journal, meditate on the messages you received, and observe how Astral Travel has impacted your life.

Ethics of Astral Travel:

- **Respect:** Respect the free will of other beings, not interfering with their experiences or energies.
- **Responsibly:** Use Astral Travel responsibly, avoiding invading the privacy of others or causing any kind of harm.

Astral Travel is a powerful tool to expand your consciousness, accelerate your spiritual growth, and connect with the vastness of the universe. With the guidance of the Arcturians, you can safely explore the astral plane, access hidden knowledge, and integrate the learnings from this transformative journey into your life.

Chapter 26
Arcturian Communication

Arcturian Communication is a profoundly transformative experience that opens the channels of human consciousness to a direct connection with universal wisdom. Through this practice, it is possible to interact with the masters of Arcturus, receiving messages, healing, and guidance to illuminate your evolutionary journey. These interdimensional beings, known for their compassionate energy and high vibration, share insights that transcend linear understanding, allowing for a significant expansion of intuition and perception. The connection with the Arcturians is not limited to words or symbols; it manifests as an energetic flow that inspires, balances, and awakens the highest potential of each being.

To establish this communication, it is essential to cultivate a state of receptivity and inner attunement. Intuition, as the most direct channel, must be strengthened by practices that silence mental noise and connect the individual to their spiritual essence. During meditation, for example, it is possible to visualize the presence of the Arcturians, feel their loving energy, and open oneself to receive their messages. In addition, dreams are a rich pathway for this interaction, as in them the conscious mind relaxes and allows access to higher dimensions. Messages can arrive in the form of images, symbols, or striking emotions, bringing clear answers and directions for personal growth.

Channeling is also a powerful tool for communicating with the Arcturians. Whether through writing, speaking, or artistic expression, the act of channeling involves allowing their energy to flow as a means of transmitting their messages. For those who feel called to this practice, preparation is crucial: a clear intention, an open heart, and an energetically protected space are fundamental to ensure that communication is authentic and luminous. At the same time, signs in everyday life - such as synchronicities, repeating numbers, or messages in music - are subtle reminders of the Arcturian presence, encouraging mindfulness and continuous connection.

Strengthening the bond with the Arcturians requires practice and dedication. Meditating regularly, invoking their presence with gratitude, and using tools like specific crystals can deepen this relationship. When receiving their messages, it is vital to trust your intuition and use discernment to ensure that the information resonates with your inner truth. This communication is not just a dialogue, but an invitation to live in alignment with cosmic wisdom, allowing Arcturian guidance to illuminate every aspect of your existence. Through this transformative exchange, Arcturian Communication becomes a source of healing, inspiration, and spiritual evolution.

The Arcturians, beings of light who vibrate in higher dimensions, wish to communicate with us, sharing their wisdom, love, and guidance to assist in our evolutionary journey. They communicate through various channels, such as intuition, dreams, meditation, channeling, and even through subtle signs in everyday life. Arcturian Communication is a two-way street, where you can send your questions, requests, and gratitude, and receive answers, insights, and healing.

Opening the Channels of Intuition:
Intuition is the language of the soul, the subtle voice that guides us and connects us with inner wisdom. To communicate with the Arcturians, it is essential to develop your intuition, learning to recognize your inner voice and trust its messages. The Arcturians assist us in this process, sending signs and messages that strengthen our intuition and connect us with cosmic wisdom.

Forms of Arcturian Communication:
- **Intuition:** Pay attention to your feelings, thoughts, and sudden "insights". Intuition manifests as an inner voice, a hunch, a sense of certainty, or creative inspiration. Trust

your intuition, it is the most direct channel of communication with the Arcturians.
- **Dreams:** Dreams are portals to other dimensions, where we can receive messages from the Arcturians, visit Arcturus and interact with its inhabitants. Pay attention to your dreams, write them down when you wake up, and look for symbols, messages, and emotions that may contain Arcturian wisdom.
- **Meditation:** Meditation calms the mind, silences the ego, and opens space for communication with the Arcturians. During meditation, you can visualize the Arcturians, send them questions, and receive their answers through images, thoughts, or feelings.
- **Channeling:** Channeling is the process of receiving messages from the Arcturians through writing, speaking, or other forms of expression. If you feel called to channel, prepare yourself through meditation, connection with the Arcturians, and the pure intention to serve as a channel of light.
- **Signs:** The Arcturians can send subtle signs in everyday life, such as repeating numbers, songs that touch your heart, unexpected encounters, or synchronicities that catch your attention. Be aware of the signs, they may contain important messages from the Arcturians.

Strengthening the Connection with the Arcturians:
- **Meditation:** Meditate regularly, visualizing the Arcturians and sending them love and gratitude.
- **Invocation:** Invoke the presence of the Arcturians in your moments of stillness, requesting their guidance and assistance.
- **Crystals:** Use crystals that facilitate communication with the Arcturians, such as amethyst, clear quartz, and selenite.
- **Gratitude:** Express gratitude to the Arcturians for their presence and guidance in your life.

Receiving Messages with Clarity:
- **Intention:** Set the intention to receive messages from the Arcturians with clarity and discernment.
- **Trust:** Trust your intuition and your ability to receive messages.
- **Discernment:** Use discernment to evaluate the messages you receive, making sure they resonate with your heart and your inner truth.

Arcturian Communication is a journey of opening to cosmic wisdom, an opportunity to connect with beings of light who wish to assist in your evolution. By developing your intuition, strengthening your connection, and trusting your ability to receive messages, you will be opening the doors to deep and transformative communication with the Arcturians, receiving guidance, healing, and inspiration to walk your path of light.

Chapter 27
Healing with Masters

The connection with the Arcturian Ascended Masters is a portal to access universal wisdom, deep healing, and unconditional love. These enlightened beings, who have transcended the limitations of three-dimensional existence, are dedicated to assisting humanity on its evolutionary journey. Their presence is like a beacon that illuminates the path of those who seek to align with their divine essence, promoting inner transformations that reflect in the external world. The Arcturian Masters, with their compassionate and vibrationally elevated energy, offer guidance to heal emotional wounds, harmonize energies, and awaken inner wisdom, helping each individual to manifest their highest potential.

Among the best-known masters, Juliano stands out for his connection with Gaia Consciousness, guiding in harmonization with the energies of the Earth and in cultivating a deep spiritual connection with the planet. Sananda, who embodies Christ consciousness, guides seekers in the practice of unconditional love, compassion, and forgiveness, fundamental pillars for spiritual growth and unity. Metatron, in turn, acts as a guardian of cosmic wisdom, helping in the activation of DNA, in the understanding of sacred geometry, and in the expansion of consciousness. Each master has a unique role, and the connection with them can be personalized according to the needs and intentions of those who invoke them.

To establish communication with these masters, it is essential to create a space of receptivity and reverence. Meditation is a powerful tool to tune in to their presence, allowing their energy to manifest clearly and transformatively. Visualizing the desired master, invoking their name with gratitude, or creating a dedicated altar are practices that help strengthen the connection. Mantras and affirmations can also be used to attune to their vibration, promoting a state of energetic alignment that facilitates the reception of their messages. It is important to remember that this interaction occurs in a subtle and loving field, where intuition serves as a bridge to understand and integrate the teachings received.

The Arcturian Masters not only share their wisdom but also inspire practical and reflective actions in everyday life. Their teachings encourage the practice of virtues such as forgiveness, compassion, and harmony, essential values for those who seek to live in alignment with high spiritual principles. Reflecting on their messages and incorporating them into daily decisions creates a cycle of continuous learning and evolution. Thus, the journey with the Ascended Masters is not limited to individual seeking; it becomes a contribution to the collective awakening of humanity, bringing light, balance, and purpose to the world.

The Arcturian Ascended Masters are beings who have reached a high level of spiritual evolution, transcending the limitations of the third dimension and dedicating themselves to loving service to humanity. They are like beacons of light that illuminate the path of ascension, sharing their wisdom and compassion to assist those who seek healing, self-knowledge, and connection with the Divine. Through connection with the Arcturian Masters, you can receive guidance, healing, and inspiration to walk your evolutionary path with more clarity, purpose, and love.

Knowing the Arcturian Masters:
- **Juliano:** Juliano is an Arcturian ascended master known for his wisdom, compassion, and dedication to planetary healing. He is a loving guide who assists in connecting with Gaia Consciousness, harmonizing telluric energies, and co-creating a sustainable future.
- **Sananda:** Sananda is the Christic consciousness that manifests through various avatars, including Jesus Christ.

He represents unconditional love, compassion, and forgiveness, guiding humanity towards ascension and unity.
- **Metatron:** Metatron is an archangel and ascended master known for his cosmic wisdom and connection to sacred geometry. He assists in DNA activation, consciousness expansion, and understanding the mysteries of the universe.

Invoking the Presence of the Masters:

To connect with the Arcturian Masters, you can:
- **Meditate:** Meditate by visualizing the master you wish to contact, feeling their presence and opening yourself to receive their messages.
- **Invoke:** Invoke the master by name, with reverence and gratitude, requesting their presence and guidance.
- **Create an altar:** Create an altar with images, crystals, and other objects that represent the master, dedicating this space to connecting with their energy.
- **Use mantras:** Use specific mantras to invoke the presence of the master and attune to their vibration.

Receiving the Teachings of the Masters:

The Arcturian Masters communicate through various channels, such as intuition, dreams, channeling, and subtle signs in everyday life. Be attentive to the messages you receive, trusting your intuition and discernment to interpret the teachings of the masters.

Integrating the Wisdom of the Masters:
- **Study:** Study the teachings of the Arcturian Masters, deepening your knowledge of spirituality, healing, and ascension.
- **Reflection:** Reflect on the teachings of the masters, applying them in your daily life and seeking to integrate their wisdom into your actions and decisions.
- **Practice:** Practice the techniques and teachings of the masters, cultivating unconditional love, compassion, forgiveness, and wisdom in your daily life.

The Arcturian Ascended Masters are loving guides who accompany us on our evolutionary journey, offering their wisdom, healing, and inspiration. By connecting with the masters, you will be opening your heart to the light, love, and wisdom of the universe, walking the path of ascension with more clarity, purpose, and joy.

Chapter 28
Healing with Angels

Arcturian Angel Healing is an experience that unites the vibrational wisdom of the Arcturians with the celestial purity of angels, creating a powerful synergy of love, protection, and transformation. This practice combines the advanced energy technology of the Arcturians with the divine and compassionate energy of angels, promoting healing on physical, emotional, mental, and spiritual levels. By opening yourself to this connection, you allow yourself to be enveloped in wings of light, feeling the peace, serenity, and acceptance that these angelic beings provide, while Arcturian wisdom amplifies and integrates the healing energy, raising your vibration and harmonizing your energy fields.

The partnership between the Arcturians and the angels transcends the limits of the known, with the Arcturians using their ability to create energy portals that facilitate interaction with the celestial realms. Through these portals, angels bring their loving energy directly to the human field, assisting in healing and spiritual evolution. For example, Archangel Michael, with his protective strength, helps to cut negative energy ties and create a shield of light around you, while Archangel Raphael offers physical and emotional healing, regenerating worn out energies and promoting balance. These celestial masters work in harmony with the Arcturians to create a unique experience of upliftment and transformation.

To connect with this energy, the first step is to set a clear and sincere intention. Prayer and invocation, accompanied by conscious visualization, help to establish a bridge between your essence and the angelic realms. During meditation, you can visualize the presence of angels around you, feeling their luminous wings enveloping you in protection and healing. Their messages can come as feelings, images, or even direct insights, offering guidance and comfort on your journey. This practice not only promotes healing, but also strengthens your connection to divine love and inspires actions aligned with compassion and inner peace.

By integrating the blessings of angels into your life, you open yourself to continuous transformation. Giving thanks for their presence and trusting in their guidance creates a deeper and more lasting bond with these beings of light. Furthermore, by following the example of unconditional love and service of the angels, you too can be a source of light to others, spreading the healing energies you have received. Arcturian Angel Healing is not just a process of individual elevation, but an experience that connects your essence to the universal flow of love and harmony, illuminating your path and positively impacting everyone around you.

The Arcturians, with their deep connection to the higher realms, recognize angels as beings of light who emanate the unconditional love of the Creator, dedicating themselves to the protection, healing, and guidance of humanity. Arcturian Angel Healing combines the technological and vibrational wisdom of the Arcturians with the purity and unconditional love of angels, creating a powerful synergy that amplifies healing, harmonizes energy fields, and raises vibration. It is a journey of connection with the celestial realm, where you open yourself to receive the blessings, healing, and protection of angels, guided by the wisdom and compassion of the Arcturians.

Understanding the Synergy between Arcturians and Angels:

The Arcturians and the angels work together to assist humanity on its evolutionary journey. The Arcturians, with their advanced technology and knowledge of energy, create portals and channels that facilitate connection with the angelic realms, amplifying the healing and protective energy of the angels.

Angels, in turn, bring purity, unconditional love, and divine wisdom, guiding and inspiring humanity on its path of ascension.

Invoking the Presence of Angels:

- **Intention:** Set the intention to connect with the angels and receive their healing and protection.
- **Prayer:** Offer a sincere prayer, expressing your desire to connect with the angels and receive their blessings.
- **Invocation:** Invoke the angels by name, such as Archangel Michael, Archangel Raphael, Archangel Gabriel, etc., requesting their presence and assistance.
- **Visualization:** Visualize the angels around you, enveloping you in their wings of light and filling you with their loving energy.
- **Meditation:** Meditate with the intention of connecting with the angels, feeling their presence and receiving their messages.

Working with Angels in Healing:

- **Physical Healing:** Invoke the angels to assist in the healing of illnesses, pains, and physical imbalances. Visualize angelic energy flowing through your body, promoting regeneration and well-being.
- **Emotional Healing:** Ask the angels to help you release negative emotions, traumas, and limiting patterns. Feel the love and compassion of the angels soothing your heart and healing your emotional wounds.
- **Mental Healing:** Ask the angels to help you calm your mind, free yourself from negative thoughts, and cultivate inner peace. Feel the clarity and serenity that emanate from the angels filling your mind.
- **Spiritual Protection:** Invoke the protection of angels to protect yourself from negative energies, dense influences, and psychic attacks. Visualize yourself enveloped in a shield of angelic light, feeling safe and protected.
- **Guidance:** Ask the angels to guide you in your decisions, show you the way, and inspire you on your evolutionary

journey. Trust the wisdom and intuition that the angels bring you.

Integrating the Blessings of Angels:
- **Gratitude:** Express gratitude to the angels for their presence, healing, and protection.
- **Trust:** Trust the wisdom and love of angels, allowing them to guide you in your life.
- **Service:** Put your gifts and talents at the service of others, inspired by the love and compassion of angels.

Arcturian Angel Healing is a journey of connection with the celestial realm, where you open yourself to receive the love, healing, and protection of angels. By invoking their presence, working with them in healing, and integrating their blessings into your life, you will be walking a path of light, guided by the wisdom of the Arcturians and supported by the unconditional love of angels.

Chapter 29
Healing with Animals

Arcturian Animal Healing is a deep reconnection with the animal kingdom, allowing access to its ancestral wisdom and the powerful healing energy that they share with humanity. This practice unites the sensitivity and knowledge of the Arcturians with the spiritual strength of power animals, promoting a state of balance, harmony, and transformation. Each animal, with its unique characteristics, carries a symbolic and energetic meaning, serving as a guide, protector, and healer. Through this interaction, you can integrate valuable lessons, find strength in challenging moments, and awaken dormant aspects of your consciousness.

Power animals are not just physical beings, but spiritual manifestations that reflect essential qualities of their species. The eagle, for example, inspires vision and elevation, helping to expand perspective and find clarity in complex situations. The wolf represents intuition and the ability to work in harmony with the group, while the butterfly symbolizes transformation and renewal, encouraging acceptance of life's changes. The Arcturians, with their advanced vibrational technology, help create an energy field that amplifies the connection with these animal guides, enhancing healing and allowing for a deeper and more meaningful interaction.

To access the presence of power animals, it is essential to enter a state of stillness and receptivity. During meditation, visualize yourself in a natural environment that resonates with you, such as a forest or a mountain. Allow the power animals to reveal themselves spontaneously, trusting your intuition to interpret their messages and energy. Sometimes these animals may appear in dreams, in recurring images, or in unexpected encounters in everyday life. Paying attention to these signs and honoring their presence is the first step to working with them consciously.

The teachings of power animals can be integrated into everyday life in a number of ways. Reflecting on their qualities and how to apply them to your own challenges and aspirations promotes personal growth. Furthermore, observing nature and learning from the behavior of animals in their habitat reinforces the connection to the cycle of life and the interdependence of all forms of existence. Gratitude is fundamental in this process, recognizing animals as spiritual partners on your evolutionary journey.

This practice is not just a personal experience, but also an invitation to live in harmony with nature and recognize the vital role of animals in planetary balance. Working with power animals, guided by the wisdom of the Arcturians, strengthens your connection to the universe, broadens your perception, and inspires a deep respect for life. Arcturian Animal Healing is, above all, a journey of union with the natural world, where you awaken to the interconnectedness of all things and find the transformative power that resides within you and around you.

The Arcturians, with their deep reverence for life in all its forms, recognize animals as beings of light who share the journey on Earth with us. Each animal has a unique wisdom and energy, which can help us in healing, self-knowledge, and connection with nature. Arcturian Animal Healing combines the ancestral wisdom of power animals with the technology and compassion of the Arcturians, creating a powerful synergy that promotes healing, balance, and expansion of consciousness. It is a journey of reconnection with the animal kingdom, where you open yourself to receive the wisdom, healing, and protection of power animals, guided by the light of the Arcturians.

Understanding Power Animals:

Power animals are spirit guides that manifest in the form of animals, bringing with them the wisdom, strength, and medicine of their species. They accompany us on our journey, protecting us, teaching us, and helping us to manifest our potential. Each power animal has specific characteristics and qualities, which resonate with different aspects of our being and assist us in different areas of life.

Invoking the Presence of Power Animals:

- **Meditation:** Meditate with the intention of connecting with your power animals. Visualize yourself in a natural setting, such as a forest, beach, or mountain, and ask your power animals to show themselves to you.
- **Intuition:** Pay attention to the animals that catch your attention, be they physical animals or images of animals that appear in your dreams, meditations, or thoughts. These animals may be your power animals, bringing important messages and teachings.
- **Invocation:** Invoke the presence of your power animals, calling them by name or species. Express your gratitude for their presence and ask for their guidance and help.

Working with Power Animals in Healing:

- **Physical Healing:** Each power animal has a specific "medicine" that can aid in the healing of different diseases and physical imbalances. For example, the bear can help heal bone and muscle problems, while the butterfly can help heal respiratory diseases.
- **Emotional Healing:** Power animals can assist in the healing of traumas, fears, and emotional blocks. For example, the wolf can help overcome fear and release past traumas, while the dolphin can help heal depression and connect with joy.
- **Mental Healing:** Power animals can aid in mental clarity, focus, and concentration. For example, the eagle can assist in strategic vision and decision-making, while the owl can assist in intuition and wisdom.
- **Spiritual Development:** Power animals can assist in spiritual development, connection with nature, and expansion of consciousness. For example, the serpent can assist in transmutation and awakening the kundalini, while

the jaguar can assist in connecting with the spiritual world and the shamanic journey.

Integrating the Teachings of Power Animals:
- **Observation:** Observe the behavior of animals in nature, learning from their wisdom and intuition.
- **Contemplation:** Contemplate the qualities of your power animals, reflecting on how you can integrate these qualities into your life.
- **Gratitude:** Express gratitude to your power animals for their presence, guidance, and healing.

Arcturian Animal Healing is a journey of reconnection with animal wisdom, an opportunity to connect with the strength, intuition, and healing that power animals offer us. By invoking their presence, working with them in healing, and integrating their teachings into your life, you will be expanding your consciousness, awakening your potential, and walking a path of harmony with nature and the universe.

Chapter 30
Healing with Plants

Arcturian Plant Healing is a deep dive into the healing energy of the plant kingdom, a symphony between the ancestral wisdom of nature and the vibrational technology of the Arcturians. In this process, plants, living beings that channel the vital energy of the Earth and the cosmos, become powerful allies to promote balance and regeneration on all levels: physical, emotional, mental, and spiritual. The combination of Arcturian consciousness with the natural properties of plants enhances their therapeutic power, allowing them to act not only on the body, but also on the subtle fields of being, harmonizing it with universal vibrations.

Each plant has a unique energy signature that resonates with specific aspects of the human being. Lavender, for example, emanates a calming and stabilizing energy, ideal for reducing stress and promoting restful sleep. Rosemary, on the other hand, offers mental clarity and vitality, being a stimulus for memory and focus. The Arcturians, with their advanced technology, understand how these physical and vibrational properties interact with the chakras, meridians, and the auric field, creating an amplified healing potential when plants are used in conscious practices. This interaction reflects the principle of unity between all life forms, where the plant kingdom becomes a fundamental link for integral health.

The integration of plants into healing rituals can be done in a number of ways, each taking advantage of a specific aspect of their energy. Teas and infusions, prepared with intention and respect, release chemical and vibrational compounds from plants, promoting immediate and subtle therapeutic effects.

Aromatherapy, in turn, uses essential oils to interact with the senses and the nervous system, allowing the essence of the plant to reach the physical and emotional levels. Herbal baths and compresses are traditional forms that provide localized relief and energy balance, while elixirs and flower essences act directly on the subtle fields, bringing emotional and spiritual harmony.

To enhance these practices, it is possible to invoke the presence of the Arcturians during the preparation or use of plants. Visualizing Arcturian energy flowing to the herbs or to the healing environment amplifies their effects, allowing the synergy between vibrational technology and nature to manifest powerfully. Growing your own medicinal plants in a healing garden is also a way to connect more deeply with the energy of the plant kingdom. This act not only strengthens the relationship with nature, but also promotes a more intimate understanding of the essence of plants and their contribution to the balance of the planet.

By opening yourself to Arcturian Plant Healing, you not only benefit from its therapeutic properties, but also awaken to the interconnection between all beings. This practice invites you to harmonize with natural cycles, to listen to the silent wisdom of plants, and to recognize their presence as guides and healers. Under the loving guidance of the Arcturians, each leaf, flower, and root becomes a gateway to a higher state of consciousness, where healing and balance are reflections of your unity with life.

The Arcturians, with their deep reverence for nature, recognize the healing power of plants as a gift from Mother Earth. Plants are living beings that vibrate in harmony with the universe, absorbing the vital energy of the sun, earth, and water, and transforming it into compounds that promote healing and balance. Arcturian Plant Healing combines the ancestral wisdom of phytotherapy with the technology and consciousness of the Arcturians, creating a powerful synergy that amplifies the healing power of plants and promotes integral well-being.

The Synergy between Arcturian Healing and the Plant Kingdom:

The Arcturians, with their advanced technology, are able to identify the healing properties of plants at subtle levels, understanding their vibrations and how they interact with the human energy field. They use this wisdom to enhance the healing power of plants, creating elixirs, essences, and vibrational frequencies that amplify their therapeutic effects.

Healing Properties of Plants:

Each plant has specific healing properties, which act on different systems of the body and promote physical, emotional, and spiritual balance. Some plants and their properties:

- **Lavender:** Calming, relaxing, helps fight stress and insomnia.
- **Chamomile:** Calming, anti-inflammatory, aids in digestion and relaxation.
- **Rosemary:** Stimulating, antioxidant, improves memory and concentration.
- **Mint:** Refreshing, digestive, helps fight nausea and headaches.
- **Ginger:** Anti-inflammatory, analgesic, aids in digestion and in fighting colds and flu.
- **Aloe Vera:** Healing, anti-inflammatory, helps heal burns and wounds.

Using Plants in Arcturian Healing:

- **Teas and Infusions:** Prepare teas and infusions with the plants you wish to use, following dosage and preparation instructions.
- **Aromatherapy:** Use essential oils for inhalation, massage, or aromatherapy baths, taking advantage of the therapeutic properties of plant aromas.
- **Herbal Baths:** Prepare herbal baths to relax, purify, and energize the body.
- **Compresses:** Use plant compresses to relieve pain, inflammation, and wounds.

- **Elixirs and Essences:** Prepare elixirs and flower essences to balance emotions and promote energy healing.

Preparing Remedies with Arcturian Energy:

When preparing your remedies with plants, invoke the presence of the Arcturians and ask them to amplify the healing power of the plants. Visualize Arcturian energy flowing through the plants, enhancing their therapeutic effects.

Cultivating your Healing Garden:

Grow your own medicinal plants at home, creating a healing garden that will provide you with connection to nature, well-being, and healing. By taking care of your plants, you will also be cultivating your health and well-being.

Arcturian Plant Healing is a journey of connection with the ancestral wisdom of the plant kingdom, an opportunity to harmonize with nature and awaken inner healing. By using plants as allies in healing, guided by the wisdom of the Arcturians, you will be walking a path of well-being, balance, and expansion of consciousness.

Chapter 31
Healing for Children

The compassionate and loving energy of the Arcturians provides a unique and profound approach to caring for the well-being and development of children. This connection is characterized by an aura of serenity and balance, which promotes the integral health of the body, mind, and spirit of the little ones. Through energy harmonization, the Arcturians contribute to the emotional, mental, and spiritual development of children, enhancing their creativity and expanding their consciousness. This approach values the natural sensitivity of children, offering a path of love and protection that strengthens their bonds with the world around them and with the higher dimensions of existence.

Children are deeply connected to the energies of the universe, easily absorbing vibrations that influence their behavior and health. This receptivity makes it essential to offer them energetically balanced environments and practices that help them develop resilience in the face of emotional or external challenges. Arcturian healing methods meet these needs in an intuitive and caring way, adapting to the unique nature of each child. By using creative visualizations, interactive stories, and playful elements such as crystals and music, Arcturian healing transforms the harmonization process into an engaging and meaningful experience, while stimulating the interest and imagination of the little ones.

More than a healing practice, the connection with Arcturian energy helps to awaken the innate potential of children, encouraging the development of their intuitive and creative abilities. Through adapted techniques such as chromotherapy, healing sounds, and simple meditations, it is possible to create an environment conducive to emotional and spiritual strengthening. These practices also promote a deep sense of security and self-esteem, essential for children to grow with confidence in their abilities and sensitivity. By benefiting from this holistic approach, each child is supported in their journey of self-discovery, with a balance that resonates with the purity and joy that are their natural essence.

Children are beings of light who bring with them purity, joy, and spontaneity. Their bodies, minds, and spirits are in constant development, absorbing the energies of the environment and shaping themselves to life experiences. Arcturian Healing for Children recognizes the sensitivity and purity of the little ones, offering techniques and tools that assist in healthy development, emotional balance, and the expansion of consciousness. It is a journey of love, healing, and protection, where the Arcturians join the children, guiding them on their path of discovery and awakening their potentials.

The Sensitivity of Children:

Children are highly sensitive beings who pick up on the energies of the environment very easily. They can be affected by dense energies, negative emotions, and disharmonious environments, which can lead to emotional imbalances, learning difficulties, and health problems. Arcturian Healing for Children offers tools to protect children from negative energies, harmonize their energy fields, and promote healthy development at all levels.

Adapting Arcturian Techniques:

Arcturian healing techniques can be adapted for children, considering their age, level of understanding, and specific needs. It is important to use simple, playful, and creative language that sparks the interest and imagination of the little ones.

- **Visualization:** Use creative visualizations, such as imagining yourself playing in a magical garden with the Arcturians, flying in a spaceship, or receiving healing from beings of light.

- **Play:** Incorporate Arcturian healing techniques into play, such as crystal healing games, Arcturian symbol drawings, and stories that teach about energy and vibration.
- **Music:** Use relaxing and harmonious music to soothe children, harmonize their energies, and facilitate connection with the Arcturians.
- **Stories:** Tell stories that teach about the Arcturians, energy healing, and spiritual development, adapting the language to the understanding of children.
- **Crystals:** Use soft and colorful crystals, such as rose quartz, amethyst, and fluorite, to harmonize children's energies and promote well-being.

Healing Techniques for Children:
- **Energy Healing:** Use the laying on of hands to harmonize children's chakras, balance their subtle bodies, and remove energy blockages.
- **Chromotherapy:** Use vibrant and cheerful colors to energize and harmonize children. Ask them to visualize the colors surrounding their bodies, bringing joy, healing, and protection.
- **Healing Sounds:** Use relaxing music, nature sounds, and mantras to soothe children, harmonize their energies, and facilitate connection with the Arcturians.
- **Communication with the Arcturians:** Encourage children to communicate with the Arcturians through visualization, drawing, and intuition. Teach them to ask the Arcturians for help in times of need and to thank them for their presence and protection.

Assisting in Child Development:
- **Emotional Balance:** Arcturian Healing for Children assists in emotional balance, helping children deal with their emotions, overcome fears, and develop self-esteem.
- **Development of Consciousness:** Arcturian techniques stimulate the development of consciousness, intuition, and creativity in children, awakening their potential and expanding their perception of reality.

- **Learning:** Arcturian Healing for Children can assist in learning, improving concentration, memory, and the ability to assimilate new knowledge.
- **Health:** Arcturian techniques strengthen children's immune systems, helping to prevent and heal diseases.

Creating a Harmonious Environment:

Create a harmonious and loving environment for children where they feel safe, loved, and protected. Use Arcturian energy to purify the environment, harmonize energies, and create a space conducive to healthy development and the expansion of consciousness.

Arcturian Healing for Children is a journey of love, healing, and protection, where the Arcturians join the children, guiding them on their path of discovery and awakening their potentials. By adapting Arcturian healing techniques for the little ones, you will be contributing to the development of more conscious, loving, and harmonious human beings who will bring light and healing to the world.

Chapter 32
Healing for Couples

Love between couples is a transformative force, capable of promoting healing, growth, and a deeper connection between two souls. Arcturian energy offers a compassionate and enriching approach to relationships, allowing couples to harmonize their energies, strengthen their bonds, and face challenges with wisdom and love. Through practices that balance body, mind, and spirit, Arcturian healing helps build relationships based on authenticity, mutual respect, and genuine expression of feelings. This journey provides not only conflict resolution but also the blossoming of love in its purest and most unconditional form.

Relationships are sacred spaces of learning and evolution, in which fears and insecurities often surface, challenging partners to grow together. Through conscious communication and the cultivation of empathy, couples can overcome emotional barriers and find common ground that strengthens their union. Arcturian techniques, such as energy healing, the use of crystals, and shared meditation, create an environment of trust and harmony. These practices help dissolve blockages, heal emotional wounds, and renew connection, allowing love to flow more freely and authentically.

By integrating tools such as forgiveness, reframing past experiences, and moments dedicated to gratitude, couples can rewrite their stories into a more loving and balanced narrative. Arcturian energy assists in this process, increasing mutual understanding and promoting compassion. The result is a relationship where both partners feel seen, heard, and valued. With dedication and the use of these practices, it is possible not only to resolve daily challenges but also to create a connection so strong that it becomes a source of inspiration and support for each stage of life.

The Arcturians, with their deep understanding of love and relationships, teach us that love is a powerful force that unites souls, drives evolution, and connects us with our divine essence. Love relationships are opportunities for growth, healing, and expansion, where we can learn about ourselves, develop compassion, and manifest unconditional love. Arcturian Healing for Couples offers tools and techniques to strengthen bonds, harmonize energies, heal past wounds, and build a deeper, more loving, and lasting relationship.

Understanding the Challenges of Relationships:

Love relationships can be challenging, bringing to the surface fears, insecurities, and patterns from the past. Personality differences, divergent expectations, lack of communication, and life challenges can create conflicts and imbalances in the relationship. Arcturian Healing for Couples helps us understand the dynamics of the relationship, identify challenges, and use healing tools to strengthen the union and build a more harmonious future.

Healing Techniques for Couples:

- **Conscious Communication:** Authentic and respectful communication is the foundation of any healthy relationship. The Arcturians teach us to communicate our needs, emotions, and expectations clearly and lovingly, creating a space for open and receptive dialogue.
- **Energy Healing:** Arcturian energy healing helps harmonize the energy fields of the couple, dissolving blockages, healing emotional wounds, and strengthening the energy connection between partners.
- **Forgiveness and Compassion:** Forgiveness is essential for healing relationships. Forgiving yourself and your partner for past hurts and misunderstandings releases the dense energies that prevent love from flowing freely. Compassion allows us to understand each other's difficulties, cultivating empathy and unconditional love.

- **Reframing the Past:** Often, past traumas and patterns interfere with the dynamics of the relationship, creating conflicts and imbalances. Arcturian Healing for Couples helps us reframe the past, freeing ourselves from limiting patterns and creating a more positive and harmonious future.
- **Meditation for Couples:** Meditating together strengthens the connection, harmonizes energies, and promotes inner peace. Visualize yourselves enveloped in light, feeling love and gratitude flowing between you.
- **Crystals for Love:** Use crystals that amplify love, harmony, and connection, such as rose quartz, amethyst, and rhodochrosite. Place the crystals in the bedroom, use them in meditations, or gift each other with crystals that symbolize love and union.

Applying Healing for Couples:
- **Open Dialogue:** Create a space for open and honest dialogue where you can share your feelings, needs, and expectations without fear of judgment.
- **Quality Time:** Set aside time to connect, have fun, and strengthen your bonds.
- **Forgiveness:** Practice forgiveness, releasing past hurts and making space for love and healing.
- **Energy Healing:** Use Arcturian energy healing techniques to harmonize your energy fields and strengthen your connection.
- **Gratitude:** Express gratitude to each other for your presence, love, and support.

Arcturian Healing for Couples is a journey of love, healing, and expansion, where you come together to strengthen your bonds, harmonize energies, and build a deeper and more lasting relationship. By using Arcturian healing tools and techniques, you will be awakening the flame of unconditional love, creating a relationship that propels you toward ascension and the fulfillment of your soul purpose.

Chapter 33
Healing for Family

The family is the space where we learn the first lessons about love, coexistence, and unity, and also where we encounter the challenges that shape our emotional and spiritual journey. Arcturian energy offers a path of deep healing, assisting in the harmonization of family relationships and overcoming patterns that cross generations. Through understanding and transformation, Arcturian Healing for Family strengthens bonds, promotes forgiveness, and creates an environment of acceptance where each member can grow and evolve. This journey invites us to look at family dynamics with an open heart, allowing unconditional love to flow with greater intensity and authenticity.

Each family has a unique history, full of beliefs, values, and memories that influence relationships. Many of these influences are positive, but others can generate conflicts and imbalances. Arcturian energy helps us identify limiting patterns and ancestral traumas that affect family interactions, offering tools to heal these wounds and transform the energy of the home. Through practices such as meditating together, conscious communication, and energy harmonization, it is possible to create a space where family members feel valued, understood, and connected to each other.

By integrating forgiveness, compassion, and the cultivation of meaningful moments, the family can free itself from old hurts and strengthen its emotional foundation. Mutual support and unconditional love become essential pillars in this healing journey, allowing each individual to flourish within the family nucleus. Moreover, by working together to harmonize energy fields and overcome challenges, family bonds become stronger, creating an environment that promotes peace, joy, and evolution. Through Arcturian energy, each home can be transformed into a true refuge of light and love.

The Arcturians, with their deep understanding of human relationships, recognize the family as a fundamental nucleus for the development, learning, and evolution of the soul. The family is our first contact with the world, where we learn about love, belonging, responsibility, and sharing. However, the family can also be the scene of conflicts, misunderstandings, and dysfunctional patterns that repeat themselves over generations. Arcturian Healing for Family helps us understand family dynamics, identify ancestral patterns, and use healing tools to harmonize relationships, free ourselves from limiting patterns, and build a more loving, healthy, and harmonious family environment.

Understanding Family Dynamics:

Each family has a unique dynamic, with its own beliefs, values, and behavior patterns. Often, we inherit ancestral patterns, limiting beliefs, and traumas that repeat themselves over generations, creating conflicts and imbalances in family relationships. Arcturian Healing for Family invites us to observe family dynamics with awareness, identifying recurring patterns and using healing tools to transform these patterns and create a more harmonious family environment.

Healing Techniques for Family:
- **Conscious Communication:** Authentic and respectful communication is fundamental to family harmony. The Arcturians teach us to express our needs, emotions, and expectations clearly and lovingly, creating a space for open and receptive dialogue among family members.
- **Energy Healing:** Arcturian energy healing helps harmonize the energy fields of the family, dissolving blockages, healing emotional wounds, and strengthening the connection between family members.
- **Forgiveness and Compassion:** Forgiveness is essential for healing family relationships. Forgiving yourself and

family members for past hurts and misunderstandings releases the dense energies that prevent love from flowing freely. Compassion allows us to understand the difficulties and challenges of each family member, cultivating empathy and unconditional love.
- **Healing Ancestral Patterns:** Arcturian Healing for Family helps us identify and heal ancestral patterns that repeat themselves over generations, freeing the family from limiting beliefs, traumas, and karmas that prevent harmony and well-being.
- **Meditation for Family:** Meditating together strengthens the connection, harmonizes energies, and promotes inner peace. Visualize yourselves as a united family, enveloped in light, feeling love and gratitude flowing between you.
- **Family Constellation:** Family Constellation is a therapeutic technique that assists in understanding family dynamics, identifying ancestral patterns, and resolving conflicts. Through Family Constellation, guided by Arcturian energy, it is possible to restore the flow of love and harmony in the family.

Applying Healing for Family:
- **Family Gatherings:** Promote family gatherings with the intention of strengthening bonds, sharing moments of joy, and cultivating unity.
- **Open Dialogue:** Create a space for open and honest dialogue where each family member can express themselves freely without fear of judgment.
- **Joint Activities:** Engage in joint activities, such as games, outings, trips, and volunteer work, to strengthen bonds and create positive memories.
- **Forgiveness:** Practice forgiveness, releasing past hurts and making space for love and healing.
- **Energy Healing:** Use Arcturian energy healing techniques to harmonize the energy fields of the family and strengthen the connection.

- **Unconditional Love:** Cultivate unconditional love among family members, accepting differences, respecting individualities, and offering mutual support.

Arcturian Healing for Family is a journey of love, healing, and harmonization, where the family comes together to strengthen bonds, free themselves from ancestral patterns, and build a home of light where unconditional love, peace, and joy flourish. By using Arcturian healing tools and techniques, you will be creating a healthy and harmonious family environment that nurtures the growth, evolution, and ascension of each family member.

Chapter 34
Healing for Animals

Animals are faithful and sensitive companions who share with us the journey on Earth, bringing love, joy, and profound lessons of coexistence and respect. Arcturian energy provides a special healing path for these beings, recognizing in them a divine connection and an evolutionary purpose. Through energy harmonization and the application of adapted techniques, Arcturian Healing for Animals seeks to alleviate suffering, strengthen physical and emotional well-being, and intensify the bond between humans and animals. This approach values the uniqueness of each species, promoting comprehensive care that encompasses body, mind, and spirit.

Animals have a natural sensitivity to the energies that surround them, absorbing both positive and negative vibrations from the environment and from people nearby. This receptivity can leave them vulnerable to imbalances, manifested in behavioral, emotional, or physical changes. Through Arcturian Animal Healing, it is possible to offer them energetic support that acts on subtle levels, strengthening their immune system, harmonizing their chakras, and providing relief from trauma and fears. By using techniques such as laying on of hands, chromotherapy, and telepathic communication, humans can establish an even deeper relationship of care and trust with their animal companions.

The unconditional love that animals demonstrate inspires healing practices that also involve empathy and intuitive connection. Creating a harmonious environment, offering a healthy diet, and dedicating moments of attention and affection are actions that complement energy practices and reinforce the well-being of animals. Arcturian Animal Healing goes beyond treating discomfort; it celebrates the symbiotic relationship between humans and animals, promoting a balance that benefits both parties. With this approach, it is possible to honor the sacredness of life in all its forms, contributing to the creation of a more compassionate and harmonious world for all beings.

The Arcturians, with their deep reverence for all life forms, recognize animals as sentient beings, with souls that evolve and learn throughout their journeys. They understand the importance of the bond between humans and animals, and how this connection can bring mutual benefits to both species. Arcturian Animal Healing offers tools and techniques to promote the physical, emotional, and spiritual health of animals, alleviating their suffering, strengthening their immune system, and harmonizing their energy fields. It is a journey of love, healing, and compassion, where the Arcturians join humans to care for animals, recognizing their importance on our planet and assisting them in their evolution.

Understanding Animal Sensitivity:

Animals are sensitive beings that pick up on the energies of the environment very easily. They can be affected by dense energies, negative emotions, and disharmonious environments, which can lead to emotional imbalances, inappropriate behaviors, and health problems. Arcturian Animal Healing offers tools to harmonize the energy fields of animals, protect them from negative energies, and promote well-being on all levels.

Adapting Arcturian Techniques:

Arcturian healing techniques can be adapted for animals, considering their species, temperament, and specific needs. It is important to create a calm and safe environment where the animal feels comfortable receiving healing.

- **Laying on of Hands:** Laying on of hands is a gentle and effective technique to harmonize the chakras of animals, balance their subtle bodies, and promote relaxation. Place your hands on the animal's body, visualizing Arcturian energy flowing through you and healing the animal.

- **Distance Healing:** If the animal is agitated or does not allow touch, you can perform distance healing. Visualize the animal enveloped in Arcturian light, sending it love, healing, and harmonization.
- **Chromotherapy:** Use colors that bring calm and balance to the animal, such as green, blue, and violet. You can use colored lights, crystals, or visualization to apply chromotherapy.
- **Healing Sounds:** Use relaxing music, nature sounds, or mantras to calm the animal, harmonize its energies, and facilitate connection with the Arcturians.
- **Telepathic Communication:** Communicate telepathically with the animal, sending messages of love, healing, and tranquility. Animals are receptive to telepathic communication and can understand your thoughts and intentions.

Healing Techniques for Animals:
- **Energy Healing:** Use Arcturian energy to harmonize the animal's chakras, balance its subtle bodies, and strengthen its immune system.
- **Emotional Healing:** Help the animal release trauma, fears, and anxieties using Arcturian emotional healing techniques.
- **Physical Healing:** Assist in the healing of diseases and physical imbalances, using Arcturian energy to promote regeneration and well-being.
- **Energy Protection:** Create an energy protection shield around the animal, protecting it from negative energies and dense influences.

Caring for Animals with Love:
- **Harmonious Environment:** Create a harmonious and loving environment for the animal, where it feels safe, loved, and protected.
- **Healthy Diet:** Offer the animal a healthy and balanced diet that meets its nutritional needs.

- **Physical Exercise:** Provide the animal with opportunities to exercise, play, and connect with nature.
- **Attention and Affection:** Dedicate time and attention to your animal, showing your love and affection through petting, playing, and kind words.

Arcturian Animal Healing is a journey of love, healing, and compassion, where the Arcturians join humans to care for animals, recognizing their importance on our planet and assisting them in their evolution. By using Arcturian healing tools and techniques, you will be honoring the connection between humans and animals, contributing to the well-being of your beloved companions and co-creating a more harmonious world for all species.

Chapter 35
Healing for the Environment

The environment that surrounds us is an extension of our own energy, directly influencing our balance and well-being. Arcturian Healing for the Environment offers us tools and practices to revitalize spaces and the Earth itself, promoting a deeper connection with the planet and restoring its harmony. Arcturian energy acts as a channel of light and transformation, purifying the elements of nature, raising the vibration of spaces, and contributing to environmental regeneration. This journey invites us to take an active role as guardians of the Earth, caring for the environment we share with all living beings.

Each space, be it a natural or built environment, carries accumulated energies that can be beneficial or disharmonious. Dense energies, often resulting from negative emotions, conflicts, or environmental imbalances, affect not only the beings that inhabit the place, but also the health and mood of those who live there. Through the application of practices such as energy purification, harmonization with natural elements, and the use of sacred geometry symbols, it is possible to transform these spaces into places of peace and revitalization. Incorporating plants, crystals, and healing sounds into environments amplifies this positive energy, creating a vibrant and welcoming refuge.

The transformation of environments begins with the clear intention of raising their vibration and connecting them to the vital energy of the Earth. Simple actions, such as keeping spaces clean and organized, introducing natural elements, and practicing gratitude for the environment, can make a big difference. When we harmonize our surroundings, we also contribute to planetary balance, as each small revitalized space connects to the whole.

Through Arcturian Healing for the Environment, we become cocreators of a healthier and more sustainable world, nurturing both the nature around us and our own spirit.

The Arcturians, with their advanced ecological awareness, understand the interdependence between all living beings and the planet we inhabit. They recognize the Earth as a living, conscious, and sensitive being, which suffers from the impacts of pollution, the unbridled exploitation of natural resources, and disharmony in the collective consciousness. Arcturian Healing for the Environment invites us to assume our responsibility as guardians of the planet, using healing tools to harmonize environments, transmute dense energies, and contribute to the healing of the Earth.

Understanding the Energy of Environments:

The environments we inhabit, whether natural or man-made, have their own energy that influences our physical, emotional, and spiritual well-being. Disharmonious environments, with dense and stagnant energies, can affect our health, our mood, and our ability to thrive. Arcturian Healing for the Environment teaches us to identify and transmute these energies, creating harmonious and revitalizing spaces that promote well-being and connection with nature.

Healing Techniques for the Environment:

- **Energy Purification:** Use energy purification techniques to remove dense and stagnant energies from environments. You can use incense, smudging, crystals, sounds, or Arcturian energy itself to purify spaces.
- **Harmonization with Nature:** Bring nature indoors, using plants, flowers, stones, water, and natural elements to create harmonious and revitalizing spaces. The presence of nature connects us with the vital energy of the Earth, promoting balance and well-being.
- **Sacred Geometry:** Use sacred geometry to harmonize the energies of environments. Draw or use representations of symbols such as the Flower of Life, Metatron's Cube, and

the Golden Spiral to create harmonious and balanced spaces.
- **Chromotherapy:** Use colors that promote harmony, peace, and vitality in environments. Paint the walls with light and vibrant colors, use colorful decorative objects, and bring natural light into spaces.
- **Healing Sounds:** Use sounds that promote harmony and relaxation, such as soft music, nature sounds, and mantras. Sounds can aid in energy purification, harmonizing spaces, and raising vibration.

Applying Healing for the Environment:
- **Cleaning and Organization:** Keep environments clean and organized, removing unused objects, getting rid of clutter, and organizing spaces in a harmonious way.
- **Purification:** Purify environments regularly, using the techniques you have learned.
- **Connection with Nature:** Bring nature indoors by growing plants, creating gardens, and using natural elements in your decor.
- **Intention:** Set the intention to create harmonious and revitalizing spaces that promote well-being and connection with nature.
- **Gratitude:** Express gratitude for the vital energy of environments and for the opportunity to contribute to the healing of the planet.

Arcturian Healing for the Environment invites us to be agents of healing and transformation, harmonizing the spaces we inhabit and contributing to the healing of the planet. By using Arcturian healing tools and techniques, you will be raising the vibration of environments, transmuting dense energies, and co-creating a more harmonious and sustainable world for all beings.

Chapter 36
Healing for Businesses

Prosperity in business is a direct reflection of the harmony between purpose, ethics, and energy that sustains each enterprise. Arcturian Healing for Businesses invites you to align your professional activities with the highest values, promoting an environment where ethics, compassion, and purpose are the foundations of success. This process is not just an isolated practice, but a holistic integration that enhances your vision of success, uniting market demands with the need to create a positive impact on the world. By adopting this approach, you transform your work environment into a vibrant, productive, and inspiring space where creativity flows naturally and prosperity manifests as an organic result of your connection to a greater purpose.

To implement this vision in a practical way, it is essential to cultivate a workspace that reflects the highest spiritual and human values. The harmonization of the environment, for example, goes beyond physical aspects; it is about adjusting the energies that circulate in the place, using techniques such as energy purification with crystals, sounds, or other vibrational resources. This practice not only renews the atmosphere, but also promotes a sense of lightness and mental clarity, which benefits both individuals and the team as a whole. In addition, adopting a conscious stance towards prosperity means recognizing that abundance arises as a result of clear intentions, ethical decisions, and a genuine commitment to the greater good, aligning each step taken in the business with universal principles.

At the heart of this transformation is the appreciation of the people who are part of your business journey. When employees feel respected, motivated, and aligned with the organization's purpose, the collective impact is amplified. This requires a conscious effort to strengthen authentic communication, dissolve conflicts, and foster a spirit of collaboration that transcends individual interests. This approach creates a powerful synergy, where each team member perceives their role as part of a harmonious and sustainable whole. With Arcturian guidance, this spiritual integration into the business world not only promotes prosperity, but also brings a deep sense of fulfillment and contribution, aligning your actions with the principles that truly matter.

The Arcturians, with their holistic view of success, understand that prosperity in business goes beyond financial profit. For them, true success manifests when work is aligned with soul purpose, contributes to the well-being of the community, and develops with ethics, responsibility, and respect for everyone involved. Arcturian Healing for Businesses invites us to integrate spirituality into the professional world, using healing tools to create a harmonious work environment, attract prosperity, strengthen the team, and build prosperous businesses aligned with the greater good.

Integrating Spirituality into Business:

Often the business world is seen as a competitive and materialistic environment, where the pursuit of profit overrides human values and ethics. Arcturian Healing for Businesses invites us to question this view, bringing spirituality to the center of our professional activities. By integrating ethics, compassion, collaboration, and purpose into our businesses, we create a more harmonious, prosperous, and sustainable work environment where everyone involved feels valued and contributes to the success of the enterprise.

Healing Techniques for Businesses:
- **Harmonization of the Work Environment:** Use energy purification techniques to remove dense and stagnant energies from the work environment. You can use incense, crystals, sounds, or Arcturian energy itself to purify and

harmonize the space, creating a lighter, more productive, and inspiring environment.
- **Prosperity and Abundance:** Use the law of attraction and visualization to attract prosperity and abundance to your business. Visualize your business thriving, your customers satisfied, and abundance flowing in all areas of your business.
- **Team Strengthening:** Promote unity, collaboration, and team spirit among your employees. Create a work environment where everyone feels respected, valued, and motivated to contribute to the success of the business. Use Arcturian Healing for Businesses to harmonize interpersonal relationships, dissolve conflicts, and promote authentic communication.
- **Ethics and Purpose:** Define the mission, vision, and values of your business, aligning them with your soul purpose and the greater good. Build a business that contributes to society, respects the environment, and promotes human and spiritual development.
- **Conscious Decision Making:** Use intuition, meditation, and connection with the Arcturians to make conscious decisions aligned with the purpose of your business. Trust your inner wisdom and follow the guidance of the Arcturians to make decisions that benefit everyone involved.

Applying Healing for Businesses:
- **Create a Sacred Space:** Create a sacred space in your work environment where you can connect with Arcturian energy, meditate, relax, and recharge your energies.
- **Purification:** Purify the work environment regularly, removing dense and stagnant energies.
- **Visualization:** Visualize your business thriving, your customers satisfied, and abundance flowing in all areas.
- **Communication:** Promote authentic and respectful communication among team members.

- **Ethics:** Act with ethics, responsibility, and respect for everyone involved in your business.
- **Gratitude:** Express gratitude for the success of your business, for your customers, employees, and for all the opportunities that life offers you.

Arcturian Healing for Businesses invites us to build prosperous and conscious businesses that contribute to the well-being of humanity and the planet. By integrating spirituality into the professional world, using healing tools and following the guidance of the Arcturians, you will be creating a business that brings you fulfillment, abundance, and the satisfaction of contributing to a better world.

Chapter 37
Planetary Healing and Ascension

Humanity is immersed in a moment of profound transformation, where each individual is invited to recognize their connection to the cosmos and their role in raising the planet's vibration. Arcturian Planetary Healing and Ascension proposes an integrated approach, where healing energy and universal wisdom unite to propel Earth and its inhabitants to a new frequency of consciousness. This process transcends individual and social barriers, promoting a collective awakening that aligns with universal harmony, inner peace, and global unity. Every thought, action, and positive intention contributes to this journey of planetary evolution, becoming a point of light that illuminates the path to a new era of balance and unconditional love.

The current scenario, marked by climate change, social challenges, and existential crises, reflects the urgent need for a reassessment of the foundations that sustain humanity. Planetary ascension is not just an energetic phenomenon, but a call to collective responsibility. Raising the vibration requires abandoning limiting patterns and cultivating actions aligned with universal values of respect and sustainability. Arcturian energy, with its high frequency, acts as a bridge for this transition, helping humanity overcome emotional blocks, fears, and resistance, while driving the integration of new perspectives. This elevation of consciousness is essential for us to build a more connected and compassionate reality.

Contributing to the ascension of the planet is both a personal and collective task. Practices such as meditation, connection with nature, and reflection on life's purpose are essential tools to align our energies with higher frequencies.

Through Arcturian healing, we are guided to unlock our divine potential and act as catalysts for transformation. Earth, as a living organism, responds to the love, gratitude, and intention of its inhabitants. By adopting practices that promote sustainability, collaboration, and compassion, we create a positive impact that resonates not only in our immediate surroundings, but also in the cosmic web that connects all beings. This is the essence of a new era of light, which arises from the union between ancestral wisdom and spiritual evolution.

The Arcturians, with their advanced cosmic consciousness, observe Earth and humanity with love and compassion, guiding us towards planetary ascension. Ascension is an evolutionary process that raises the vibration of the planet and humanity, expanding consciousness, awakening divine potential, and leading us to a new era of light and harmony. It is a journey of profound transformation that affects all aspects of life, from the individual to the collective, propelling us to a higher reality, where love, peace, and unity prevail.

Understanding Planetary Ascension:

Planetary ascension is a process that has been underway for millennia, but has intensified in recent decades. Earth and humanity are undergoing a profound energetic transformation, which manifests itself on several levels:

- **Raising Vibration:** The vibratory frequency of the planet is rising, propelling humanity towards a more expanded consciousness and connected to the universe.
- **Awakening of Consciousness:** More and more people are awakening to their true divine nature, questioning old beliefs and seeking a deeper meaning for their lives.
- **Planetary Changes:** We are experiencing climate change, natural disasters, and geological transformations that reflect the intensification of planetary energy and the need for change and adaptation.
- **Social Transformation:** Social, political, and economic structures are being challenged, opening space for new

models based on collaboration, social justice, and sustainability.

Challenges of Ascension:

Planetary ascension is a challenging process that invites us to confront our fears, insecurities, and limiting patterns. The intensification of planetary energy can bring to the surface repressed emotions, conflicts, and resistance to change. It is important to maintain calm, confidence, and connection with your Higher Self during this process, seeking support in Arcturian healing and spiritual practices that bring you balance and inner peace.

How Arcturian Healing Helps in Ascension:

Arcturian Healing offers tools and techniques that assist in the process of planetary ascension, both individually and collectively:

- **Raising Vibration:** Arcturian healing techniques raise individual and collective vibration, facilitating adaptation to the planet's new energy frequencies.
- **Emotional Healing:** Arcturian emotional healing helps in the release of traumas, fears and emotional blocks, allowing humanity to free itself from the past and embrace the future with more lightness and confidence.
- **Expansion of Consciousness:** Arcturian techniques expand consciousness, awakening divine potential and connecting humanity with cosmic wisdom.
- **Healing the Planet:** Arcturian planetary healing harmonizes telluric energies, purifies ecosystems and promotes ecological balance, assisting in the healing of the Earth and the creation of a sustainable future.
- **Unity and Collaboration:** Arcturian Healing promotes unity and collaboration among human beings, inspiring the creation of a new society based on love, compassion, and social justice.

Contributing to Planetary Ascension:

- **Raise your Vibration:** Cultivate positive thoughts and emotions, practice meditation, connect with nature, and

use other techniques to raise your vibration and contribute to raising the planet's vibration.
- **Heal your Wounds:** Free yourself from traumas, limiting beliefs, and patterns from the past that prevent you from moving forward on your evolutionary journey.
- **Expand your Consciousness:** Question your beliefs, seek new knowledge, and open yourself to new perspectives and realities.
- **Connect with your Higher Self:** Strengthen your connection with your Higher Self, seeking guidance and inspiration for your journey.
- **Collaborate with the Healing of the Planet:** Adopt sustainable practices, take care of nature, promote peace and inspire others to join this journey of transformation.

Arcturian Planetary Healing and Ascension invites us to actively participate in the creation of a new era of light, where humanity awakens to its true divine nature and co-creates a future of peace, consciousness, and unity. Trust the wisdom of the Arcturians, surrender to the flow of life, and allow the loving energy of the universe to guide you on your journey of ascension.

Chapter 38
Awakening of Consciousness

Embark on a journey of self-discovery and expansion with the Arcturian Awakening of Consciousness, a transformative process that frees you from the illusions of limited reality and connects you with your true divine essence. Imagine yourself opening your eyes to a new reality, where perception expands, intuition sharpens, and connection with the universe intensifies. In this chapter, we will explore the profound transformation of the awakening of consciousness, understanding the stages of this process, the challenges to be overcome, and how Arcturian energy can help in this journey of self-knowledge and spiritual evolution.

The awakening of consciousness is a call to transcend the limitations of the ego, free yourself from limiting beliefs, and connect with the wisdom, love, and peace that reside within you. It is a gradual process of expanding perception, where you become more aware of yourself, others, and the universe around you. The Arcturians, with their wisdom and compassion, guide you in this process, helping you to awaken to your true divine nature and manifest your unlimited potential.

Stages of the Awakening of Consciousness:

The awakening of consciousness is an individual journey, with its own nuances and rhythms for each person. However, some common steps can be observed in this process:

1. **Questioning:** You begin to question the beliefs and values that have been taught to you, seeking a deeper meaning for life and questioning the nature of reality.

2. **Search for Knowledge:** you are attracted to spiritual knowledge, philosophies and practices that expand your worldview and connect you with your inner essence.
3. **Self-knowledge:** You dedicate yourself to self-knowledge, exploring your emotions, thoughts and behaviors, seeking to understand your patterns and free yourself from limiting conditioning.
4. **Inner Healing:** You begin a process of inner healing, releasing traumas, emotional wounds and limiting beliefs that prevent you from living fully.
5. **Expansion of Consciousness:** Your perception of reality expands, you become more intuitive, compassionate and connected with the universe.
6. **Connection with the Higher Self:** You strengthen your connection with your Higher Self, receiving guidance, inspiration and strength to walk your evolutionary path.
7. **Loving Service:** You feel inspired to serve others, sharing your gifts and talents to contribute to the healing of the planet and humanity.

Awakening Challenges:

The awakening of consciousness can bring challenges, such as:

- **Ego Resistance:** The ego, attached to its limited identity, can resist the awakening process, creating fears, insecurities, and doubts.
- **Internal Conflicts:** Confrontation with limiting beliefs and patterns from the past can generate internal conflicts and emotional challenges.
- **Changes in Life:** The awakening of consciousness can lead to significant changes in your life, such as a career change, the end of relationships, or the search for new paths.
- **Loneliness:** You may feel alone on your journey, as not everyone around you understands or shares your spiritual quest.

How Arcturian Energy Helps in Awakening:

The Arcturians, with their wisdom and compassion, assist in the process of awakening consciousness:

- **Raising Vibration:** Arcturian energy raises your vibration, facilitating the expansion of consciousness and connection with your Higher Self.
- **Energy Healing:** Arcturian energy healing removes blockages, harmonizes the chakras and balances the subtle bodies, assisting in inner healing and the release of limiting patterns.
- **Expansion of Consciousness:** The Arcturians use techniques and tools to expand your consciousness, helping you to transcend the limitations of the ego and connect with your true nature.
- **Guidance and Support:** The Arcturians offer guidance and support during the awakening process, helping you navigate the changes and challenges that arise on your journey.

The awakening of consciousness is a journey of self-discovery and liberation, where you connect with your true divine essence and manifest your unlimited potential. Trust the wisdom of the Arcturians, surrender to the flow of life, and allow the loving energy of the universe to guide you on your journey of awakening.

Chapter 39
Soul Purpose

Soul purpose is the essence that guides your existence, a unique calling that resonates deeply within you, directing your actions towards personal fulfillment and positive impact on the world. Discovering it means diving into your true nature, recognizing your gifts, talents and the unique way you can contribute to the greater good. This journey of self-discovery is not just a path of individual fulfillment, but also a link that connects you to the universal web of life, where each step towards purpose strengthens collective harmony and elevates the energy of the planet. By aligning with this mission, you experience a sense of meaning and fulfillment that transcends the limitations of everyday life.

Identifying soul purpose requires a conscious process of introspection and openness. It can manifest itself in various ways, such as a desire to serve others, create something transformative, or simply live with authenticity and joy. Connecting with your intuition is fundamental in this process, as it acts as an inner guide, pointing out the directions that most resonate with your essence. Meditation and inner silence are powerful practices that allow access to the wisdom of the soul, while exploring interests and talents helps to reveal what truly inspires and motivates you. The Arcturians, with their compassionate and guiding energy, offer support during this journey, helping to bring clarity and confidence amidst uncertainties.

Living your soul purpose is an act of courage and authenticity. It is necessary to overcome fears, insecurities and limiting beliefs that may arise along the way, recognizing them as opportunities for growth and transformation. Perseverance in the face of challenges and commitment to your inner truth are crucial elements to manifest your mission. When you embody your purpose in your life, every action becomes an expression of your highest essence, creating an impact that inspires and transforms those around you. This deep connection with your soul brings not only personal fulfillment, but also a significant contribution to the world, strengthening the bonds of love, compassion and unity that sustain humanity.

The Arcturians, with their deep understanding of the human soul, teach us that each being has a unique and special purpose to fulfill on Earth. Soul purpose is the reason you are here, the mission your soul chose to accomplish in this incarnation. It is like an internal compass that guides you towards fulfillment, happiness and wholeness. Connecting with soul purpose brings meaning to life, awakens passion, drives action and connects you with your true essence.

Unraveling your Soul Purpose:

Soul purpose manifests itself in different ways for each person. It may be related to your profession, your relationships, your creativity, your service to others, or any other area of life that brings you fulfillment and allows you to express your gifts and talents. To unravel your soul purpose, the Arcturians invite us to undertake a journey of self-knowledge, connecting with inner wisdom and opening ourselves to the guidance of the universe.

Techniques to Discover Your Purpose:

- **Intuition:** Your intuition is the compass that guides you towards your soul purpose. Pay attention to your feelings, your "insights" and the synchronicities that arise in your life. What brings you joy, enthusiasm and passion? What activities make you lose track of time? Your intuition will show you the way.
- **Meditation:** Meditation calms the mind, silences the ego and opens space for connection with your soul. Meditate with the intention of connecting with your soul purpose, asking questions like: "What is my mission in this life?"

"What are my gifts and talents?" "How can I contribute to the world?"
- **Self-knowledge:** Dedicate yourself to self-knowledge, exploring your values, your passions, your talents and your abilities. Recognize your strengths and weaknesses, your dreams and aspirations. The more you know yourself, the more clarity you will have about your soul purpose.
- **Connection with the Arcturians:** Invoke the presence of the Arcturians, requesting their guidance and assistance in discovering your soul purpose. The Arcturians can offer you insights, messages and signs that guide you on your journey.
- **Experimentation:** Try different activities, explore your interests and follow your curiosity. Experimentation allows you to discover your talents, awaken your passions and find the path that resonates with your soul.

Living Your Purpose:

Once you discover your soul purpose, it's time to live it with passion and authenticity. Incorporate your purpose into your actions, decisions and relationships. Express your gifts and talents with joy, contributing to the world and making a difference in people's lives.

Challenges and Obstacles:

The journey towards soul purpose can present challenges, such as:
- **Fears and Insecurities:** Fear of failure, rejection or judgment can prevent you from following your soul purpose.
- **Limiting Beliefs:** Limiting beliefs about yourself, your potential and your abilities can block the fulfillment of your purpose.
- **Distractions:** The distractions of everyday life, responsibilities and external pressures can take you off your path.

Overcoming Challenges:
- **Confidence:** Trust yourself, your talents and the guidance of the universe.
- **Self-knowledge:** Identify and free yourself from limiting beliefs and self-sabotaging patterns.
- **Focus:** Stay focused on your purpose, prioritizing your actions and dedicating time and energy to fulfilling your mission.
- **Persistence:** Be persistent on your journey, overcoming obstacles and learning from challenges.

Soul purpose is a call to manifest your life mission, expressing your gifts and talents with passion and authenticity. By connecting with your purpose, you will be living in alignment with your soul, contributing to the world and fulfilling your maximum potential. Trust the wisdom of the Arcturians, follow your intuition and embrace the journey of discovering and fulfilling your soul purpose.

Chapter 40
Intuition and Inner Guidance

Intuition is an internal compass that connects you to the infinite wisdom of the universe and your own divine essence, guiding you towards decisions aligned with your purpose and a life full of meaning. This subtle connection, often ignored amidst the noise of everyday life, is a powerful tool for accessing deep insights, identifying clear paths, and navigating challenges with confidence and serenity. Cultivating this sensitivity is opening yourself to a more intimate relationship with yourself and with the spiritual forces that support you, allowing your inner voice to be a constant ally in your journey of evolution.

Recognizing intuition requires attention and practice. It manifests in a unique way for each person, whether as a hunch, a physical sensation, a vision, or a sudden thought that arises with clarity and precision. The difference between intuition and the voices of the ego lies in the tranquility it transmits: while the ego shouts and demands, intuition whispers with conviction. Strengthening this communication channel requires patience and dedication, but the benefits are transformative. Meditation is an essential practice in this process, as it calms the mind, silences distractions, and creates a space where intuition can be heard more clearly.

Furthermore, connecting with your inner guide is a fundamental step in integrating intuition into your daily life. This guide is an extension of your divine essence, always present to offer loving guidance and wise counsel. To strengthen this relationship, it is essential to establish a routine of introspection, such as setting aside daily moments to invoke its presence, listen to its messages, and express gratitude. As the connection with the inner guide deepens, you realize that your decisions become more confident and fluid, as they are based on a wisdom that transcends the limitations of logical reasoning. This integration between intuition and inner guidance allows you to live in a more aligned, authentic, and harmonious way, with clarity to face challenges and enthusiasm to embrace opportunities.

The Arcturians, with their deep connection to the higher planes, recognize intuition as a direct channel of communication with the soul and the inner guide. Intuition is the subtle voice of inner wisdom, which manifests through feelings, insights, hunches, and synchronicities. It is the compass that guides us towards our soul purpose, helping us to make decisions aligned with our inner truth and to manifest our dreams.

Recognizing the Voice of Intuition:

Intuition manifests itself in different ways for each person. It can be a subtle feeling, an inner voice, an image that arises in your mind, a physical sensation, or a synchronicity that catches your attention. To recognize the voice of intuition, it is important to cultivate mindfulness, observe your thoughts and feelings without judgment, and learn to differentiate the voice of the ego from the voice of intuition.

Strengthening the Connection with the Inner Guide:

The inner guide is your connection to the Divine, your divine spark that resides in your heart. It is your inner teacher, your spiritual advisor who guides you with love and wisdom on your evolutionary journey. To strengthen the connection with your inner guide, the Arcturians teach us to:

- **Meditate:** Meditation calms the mind, silences the ego, and opens space for connection with the inner guide. Meditate with the intention of connecting with your guide, asking for guidance, healing, and inspiration.
- **Invoke:** Invoke the presence of your inner guide, calling it by the name you have given it or simply asking for its assistance and guidance.
- **Listen:** Learn to listen to the voice of your inner guide, paying attention to your feelings, insights, and intuitions.

- **Trust:** Trust the wisdom of your inner guide, even if its messages seem challenging or different from what you expected.
- **Give thanks:** Thank your inner guide for its presence, guidance, and unconditional love.

Integrating the Wisdom of Intuition and Inner Guidance:

- **Self-observation:** Cultivate self-observation, paying attention to your thoughts, feelings, and intuitions.
- **Journal:** Keep a journal to record your intuitions, insights, and messages from your inner guide.
- **Reflection:** Reflect on the messages you receive, seeking to understand their meaning and how to apply them in your life.
- **Action:** Act according to the guidance of your intuition and your inner guide, trusting in the wisdom they bring you.

Challenges and Obstacles:

- **Doubts and Fears:** The ego can create doubts and fears, making it difficult to trust intuition and the inner guide.
- **Limiting Beliefs:** Limiting beliefs about yourself and your ability to connect with inner wisdom can block intuition.
- **Distractions:** The distractions of everyday life, information overload, and lack of time to connect with yourself can hinder communication with intuition and the inner guide.

Overcoming Challenges:

- **Trust:** Cultivate trust in yourself and the wisdom of your inner guide.
- **Self-knowledge:** Identify and free yourself from limiting beliefs and self-sabotaging patterns.
- **Practice:** Practice meditation, mindfulness, and other techniques that strengthen intuition and connection with the inner guide.

Arcturian Intuition and Inner Guidance invites you to live with clarity, purpose, and confidence, guided by the wisdom that resides within you. By connecting with your intuition and your inner guide, you will be opening the doors to a more authentic, fulfilling life aligned with your true essence.

Chapter 41
Self-Healing and Self-Knowledge

Arcturian Self-Healing and Self-Knowledge reveal themselves as a direct invitation to a process of inner transformation, based on the rediscovery of the innate potential for healing and the connection with the essential wisdom that resides in each individual. This journey begins with the recognition that the healing force is not something external, but an internal manifestation that can be accessed through the harmonization of body, mind, and spirit. With the help of Arcturian energy, we are led to unlock limiting patterns, cultivate balance, and reveal our most authentic essence. This process not only awakens self-awareness but also expands our ability to safely and clearly tread a path of integral health and autonomy.

Through transformative tools such as meditation, conscious breathing, and energy healing practices, it is possible to access deep layers of our psyche and release blockages that impede the harmonious flow of vital energy. Meditation, for example, emerges as a central point of this practice, as it calms the mind and opens doors to inner guidance. Arcturian techniques, such as the use of crystals and the laying on of hands, intensify the process of energetic alignment, promoting a more intimate connection with our healing essence. Additionally, conscious breathing and creative visualization allow us to establish a bridge with the subtle energy field, projecting healing intentions that manifest physically and emotionally. All of this is strengthened by the use of positive affirmations which, by reprogramming limiting beliefs, become powerful allies in cultivating trust in our innate abilities.

By embracing responsibility for our own well-being, we transcend the passive stance towards healing and adopt a proactive vision. This commitment involves daily practices that range from conscious food choices and pleasurable physical activities to the pursuit of restful sleep and effective stress management techniques. Furthermore, contact with nature, so valued by Arcturian teachings, reinforces the feeling of oneness with the universe, providing renewing energy and balance. This awakening of the inner healer marks a return to what is essential: a life guided by self-awareness, integrity, and trust in our ability to create and sustain harmony in all dimensions of our being.

Thus, the path of self-healing and self-knowledge is established as a foundation for transformation, which not only transcends challenges but also redefines the relationship with oneself. Through regular practices and the application of Arcturian tools, each step in this process becomes an opportunity to integrate health, wisdom, and empowerment, resulting in a fuller life connected to our unlimited potential.

The Arcturians, with their profound wisdom and compassion, teach us that self-healing is a process inherent in all living beings. Our body, mind, and spirit have an innate intelligence, a natural ability to regenerate, balance, and heal themselves. Self-healing is the key to integral health, to freedom from limiting patterns, and to the manifestation of our maximum potential. Arcturian Self-Healing and Self-Knowledge invites us to access this inner wisdom, to take responsibility for our health and well-being, and to use Arcturian tools to tread a path of healing, growth, and autonomy.

The Journey of Self-Knowledge:

Self-knowledge is the basis of self-healing. By knowing ourselves deeply, we understand our patterns, beliefs, emotions, and motivations, identifying the roots of our imbalances and accessing the inner wisdom that guides us in healing. The journey of self-knowledge is a continuous process of discovery, where we explore the depths of our being, recognize our shadows, and awaken to our true essence.

Arcturian Tools for Self-Healing:
The Arcturians offer us several tools to aid in self-healing:
- **Meditation:** Meditation calms the mind, harmonizes emotions, and connects us with our inner wisdom. Through meditation, we can access the guidance of our Higher Self, receive insights about our challenges, and find paths to healing.
- **Energy Healing:** Arcturian energy healing techniques, such as the laying on of hands, chromotherapy, and the use of crystals, help to harmonize the chakras, release energy blockages, and strengthen the immune system.
- **Conscious Breathing:** Conscious breathing is a powerful tool for regulating emotions, calming the mind, and promoting relaxation. Through breathing, we can release tension, oxygenate the body, and connect with our vital energy.
- **Visualization:** Creative visualization allows us to connect with our healing capacity, imagining our body regenerating, our emotions balancing, and our mind calming.
- **Affirmations:** Positive affirmations are powerful tools to reprogram limiting beliefs and strengthen self-confidence. Repeat affirmations that express health, well-being, and empowerment, imprinting in your mind the belief in your ability to heal yourself.

Taking Responsibility for your Healing:
Self-healing is an active process that requires responsibility and commitment. Take responsibility for your health and well-being, making conscious choices that promote physical, emotional, and spiritual balance.
- **Conscious Eating:** Eat consciously, choosing nutritious foods that provide you with vitality.
- **Physical Exercise:** Move your body with joy, practicing physical activities that bring you pleasure and well-being.
- **Restful Sleep:** Get enough sleep so that your body and mind can regenerate and heal.

- **Stress Management:** Learn to manage stress using relaxation techniques, meditation, and conscious breathing.
- **Connection with Nature:** Connect with nature, absorbing the vital energy of the earth, the sun, and fresh air.

Arcturian Self-Healing and Self-Knowledge invites you to awaken the healer that resides within you, accessing the innate wisdom of your body, mind, and spirit. By knowing yourself deeply, using Arcturian tools, and taking responsibility for your healing, you will be treading a path of autonomy, empowerment, and transformation, manifesting your integral health and your unlimited potential.

Chapter 42
Forgiveness and Compassion

Arcturian Forgiveness and Compassion offer a portal to emotional and spiritual healing, guiding us in releasing accumulated suffering and building a lighter and more harmonious life. This path begins with the recognition that forgiveness is not an act of approval or forgetting the past, but rather a conscious choice to free oneself from the emotional chains that keep us tied to pain and resentment. The compassionate energy of the Arcturians helps us to look at our wounds with acceptance, transforming them into opportunities for learning and growth, while we reconnect with the unconditional love that resides in our hearts.

This process involves deep reflection on the circumstances that caused pain, accompanied by an internal decision to let go of the emotional weight associated with these experiences. Instead of clinging to anger or resentment, we learn to see beyond actions, understanding the human motivations and limitations that often lie behind conflicts. The practice of forgiveness teaches us to let go of the desire for retribution or control, replacing these impulses with empathy and a genuine desire for inner peace. This movement not only dissolves the emotional barriers that separate us from others but also promotes an energetic realignment that benefits our physical, emotional, and spiritual health.

Compassion, in turn, amplifies the impact of forgiveness, allowing us to develop a broader and more loving view of ourselves and those around us. Through it, it is possible to cultivate empathy, seeing the pains and difficulties of others as expressions of a learning journey similar to our own. When we embrace our own flaws with compassion, we open space for self-forgiveness, a vital aspect of this transformative process. By freeing ourselves from guilt and self-judgment, we reclaim our purest essence, rebuilding our relationship with ourselves on the basis of acceptance and unconditional love. In this way, forgiveness ceases to be a one-time act and becomes a state of being, a continuous flow of understanding and reconciliation that permeates our interactions and thoughts.

Walking this path of forgiveness and compassion is a gift we offer to ourselves. By freeing ourselves from the shackles of the past, we create space for a lighter life, guided by healthy relationships and deep inner peace. With the help of Arcturian practices such as meditation, positive affirmations, and empathy exercises, this journey becomes even more accessible and transformative, helping us to integrate love and harmony as central forces in our daily lives.

The Arcturians, with their profound wisdom and compassion, teach us that forgiveness is the key to freedom from suffering and to the healing of the soul. When we cling to anger, resentment, and hurt, we imprison ourselves in a cycle of pain and suffering, preventing love and peace from flourishing in our hearts. Forgiveness is an act of liberation, a gift you offer to yourself and others, opening space for healing, reconciliation, and transformation.

Understanding Forgiveness:

Forgiving does not mean forgetting or denying what happened, but rather freeing yourself from the weight of the past and choosing to move forward with lightness and compassion. It is acknowledging the pain, accepting what happened, and choosing to release anger, resentment, and hurt, replacing them with love, understanding, and inner peace.

Benefits of Forgiveness:
- **Liberation:** Forgiveness frees you from the shackles of the past, allowing you to move forward with lightness and freedom.

- **Emotional Healing:** Forgiveness heals emotional wounds, dissolving anger, resentment, and hurt that prevent you from living in peace.
- **Inner Peace:** Forgiveness brings inner peace, calming the mind and opening space for serenity and harmony.
- **Healthy Relationships:** Forgiveness promotes healthier relationships based on love, understanding, and compassion.
- **Physical Health:** Forgiveness benefits physical health, reducing stress, anxiety, and tension that can lead to illness.
- **Spiritual Evolution:** Forgiveness is an important step in the evolutionary journey, freeing you from karmic patterns and opening the way for ascension.

Cultivating Compassion:

Compassion is the ability to put yourself in another's shoes, understanding their difficulties, their pains, and their motivations. It is a feeling of empathy and unconditional love that allows us to forgive, accept, and love ourselves and others, even in the face of mistakes and imperfections.

Techniques for Forgiveness and Compassion:
- **Acknowledge the Pain:** Acknowledge the pain you are feeling, without judgment or resistance. Allow yourself to feel anger, hurt, and resentment, but do not identify with these emotions.
- **Understand:** Seek to understand the situation that caused the pain, the reasons that led the person to act that way, and the lessons you can learn from this experience.
- **Free Yourself:** Free yourself from the need to be right, to take revenge, or to punish. Choose to free yourself from the past and move forward with lightness and compassion.
- **Cultivate Empathy:** Put yourself in the other person's shoes, trying to understand their pains, their motivations, and their difficulties.
- **Affirmations:** Use affirmations that express forgiveness, compassion, and unconditional love, such as "I forgive

myself for...", "I forgive (person's name) for...", and "I open myself to love and compassion."
- **Meditation:** Meditate with the intention of cultivating forgiveness and compassion, visualizing yourself freeing yourself from the past and sending love and light to yourself and the people involved.

Forgiving Yourself:

Self-forgiveness is fundamental for healing and liberation. Often, we are harder on ourselves than we are on others, cultivating guilt, self-criticism, and self-sabotage. Forgive yourself for your mistakes, acknowledge your imperfections, and embrace yourself with love and compassion.

Arcturian Forgiveness and Compassion invites you to walk a path of healing and liberation, where you free yourself from the shackles of the past, cultivate empathy and unconditional love, and open space for inner peace and reconciliation. Trust in the wisdom of the Arcturians, surrender to the healing process, and allow forgiveness and compassion to transform your life.

Chapter 43
Gratitude and Abundance

Arcturian Gratitude and Abundance invites you to align with the infinite essence of the universe, a constant flow of love, prosperity, and fulfillment that is always available. The practice of gratitude is the key to this connection, transforming the way you perceive the world and expanding your ability to attract what you desire. Instead of focusing on what is lacking, gratitude directs your attention to the riches that already exist in your life, creating a vibrational foundation that magnetizes even more reasons to be thankful. This state of appreciation and recognition is the essence of an abundant life, as it raises your energetic frequency and unlocks paths to new opportunities.

Abundance, according to Arcturian teachings, is not limited to the material dimension; it manifests in love, health, harmonious relationships, and inner peace. Often, we are so involved with the demands and challenges of everyday life that we forget to observe the richness that surrounds us. Recognizing this abundance requires a shift in perspective, a careful look at the blessings that often go unnoticed, such as the support of loved ones, the beauty of nature, or even the small pleasures of everyday life. This practice of awareness not only brings immediate satisfaction but also expands your ability to manifest new desires.

By combining gratitude with intention, you become a conscious co-creator of your reality. Visualizing your dreams as if they have already been realized, while feeling genuine gratitude for them, creates a powerful magnetic field that attracts what you desire. Arcturian practices, such as focused meditation, positive affirmations, and the use of a gratitude journal, are effective tools for aligning thoughts and emotions with your goals. Each act of gratitude reinforces your connection to the universal source of energy, unlocking the flow of prosperity in all areas of life and strengthening your confidence in the ability to co-create a full and abundant existence.

The Arcturians, with their expanded consciousness and high vibration, understand abundance as a natural state of the universe, an infinite flow of energy, love, and prosperity available to all beings. Gratitude is the key that opens the doors to abundance, a portal that connects us with the frequency of prosperity and allows us to manifest our dreams with joy and magnetism. Arcturian Gratitude and Abundance invites us to cultivate gratitude as a way of life, to recognize the abundance that already exists in our lives, and to co-create a reality of fullness and prosperity in all areas.

Cultivating Gratitude as a State of Being:

Gratitude is not just a fleeting feeling, but a state of being, a lens through which you see the world. By cultivating gratitude, you focus on the blessings, joys, and opportunities that life offers you, raising your vibration and attracting more reasons to be thankful. Gratitude is a magnet that attracts abundance, a portal that connects you with the frequency of prosperity and happiness.

Recognizing Abundance:

Abundance manifests itself in all areas of life: love, health, relationships, prosperity, creativity, inner peace, and spiritual connection. Often, we focus on what we lack, forgetting to acknowledge and give thanks for the blessings that already exist in our lives. Arcturian Gratitude and Abundance invites us to open our eyes to the abundance that surrounds us, to recognize the wealth we already possess, and to celebrate each moment with joy and gratitude.

Manifesting Your Dreams:

Gratitude is a powerful catalyst for manifestation. When you give thanks for your dreams as if they were already reality, you align yourself with the frequency of what you desire, attracting into your life the people, situations, and opportunities that allow you to realize your dreams. Arcturian Gratitude and Abundance teaches us to use the power of gratitude, visualization, and affirmation to manifest our dreams with joy, confidence, and magnetism.

Techniques for Cultivating Gratitude and Abundance:

- **Gratitude Journal:** Keep a gratitude journal, writing down daily all the things you are grateful for. Write about the little joys, the special moments, the people you love, the opportunities that life offers you, and everything that brings you happiness and well-being.
- **Gratitude Meditation:** Meditate with the intention of cultivating gratitude, visualizing all the blessings in your life and feeling the emotion of gratitude filling your heart.
- **Abundance Affirmations:** Use affirmations that express the abundance you want to manifest in your life. Repeat phrases like "I am grateful for the abundance that flows into my life", "I attract prosperity and success with ease" and "I am a magnet for abundance".
- **Visualization:** Visualize yourself living the life you desire, surrounded by abundance, love, and happiness. Feel the emotions as if your dreams were already reality, imprinting this vibration in your energy field.
- **Actions of Gratitude:** Express your gratitude through actions, such as thanking the people you love, helping others, caring for nature, and contributing to a better world.

Arcturian Gratitude and Abundance invites us to create a flow of abundance in our lives, cultivating gratitude as a state of being, recognizing the blessings we already possess, and manifesting our dreams with joy and confidence. By connecting with the energy of gratitude, you will be opening the doors to a fuller, more prosperous and happy life, in harmony with the universe and with your divine essence.

Chapter 44
Manifestation and Co-creation

Arcturian Manifestation and Co-creation reveals the inherent power that each being possesses to shape their reality with intention, clarity, and purpose. This process begins with the understanding that creation does not occur by chance, but as a direct result of our vibrations, thoughts, and emotions. When we assume the role of conscious co-creators, we have the ability to direct these energies to align our desires with the forces of the universe, transforming dreams into tangible experiences. Arcturian energy acts as a guide in this process, amplifying our magnetism and helping us connect with the universal creative flow.

At the heart of manifestation is intention, which serves as a focal point for channeling our efforts and thoughts. A clear and specific intention acts as a compass, guiding all actions and energies in the right direction. Creative visualization complements this practice by allowing you to mentally experience the achievement of your goals, creating a deep emotional connection with what you want to manifest. This practice not only strengthens your vibration, but also communicates to the universe that you are aligned with your desires and ready to receive them.

Gratitude plays a crucial role as a catalyst in this process. By expressing gratitude for the blessings you already have and for the desires you are manifesting, you raise your vibration and attract even more abundance. This energy is potentiated by conscious action, which translates your intention into concrete movements. Manifestation is not just dreaming or wishing; it requires commitment, planning, and making decisions aligned with your goals. Thus, by integrating intention, gratitude, and action, you become an active channel for universal creative energy, co-creating a reality rich in purpose, abundance, and fulfillment.

The Arcturians, with their advanced consciousness and connection to universal laws, understand manifestation as a natural and constant process. With every thought, emotion, and action, we are creating our reality, whether consciously or unconsciously. Arcturian Manifestation and Co-creation invites us to take control of this process, becoming conscious co-creators of our reality, manifesting our dreams with clarity, intention, and alignment with our soul purpose.

Understanding the Law of Attraction:

The Law of Attraction is a universal law that states that "like attracts like". In other words, you attract into your life what you vibrate, whether in thoughts, emotions, or actions. If you vibrate at the frequency of love, you will attract love; if you vibrate at the frequency of prosperity, you will attract prosperity. Arcturian Manifestation and Co-creation teaches us to use the Law of Attraction consciously, raising our vibration, focusing on our desires, and co-creating the reality we desire.

The Power of Intention:

Intention is the driving force of manifestation. It is the energy that directs your thoughts, emotions, and actions toward your goals. Define your intentions clearly, specifying what you want to manifest in your life. The clearer and more focused your intention, the more powerful your ability to co-create your reality.

Creative Visualization:

Visualization is a powerful tool for materializing your dreams. Imagine yourself living the life you desire, feeling the emotions, sensations, and experiences as if they were already reality. Visualization sends a clear signal to the universe, attracting into your life the people, situations, and opportunities that resonate with your desires.

Gratitude as a Catalyst:

Gratitude is a powerful catalyst for manifestation. By giving thanks for your dreams as if they were already reality, you align yourself with the frequency of what you desire, attracting abundance and fulfillment into your life. Cultivate gratitude in your heart, giving thanks for the blessings you already have and for those to come.

Conscious Action:

Conscious action is fundamental to manifestation. It is not enough just to visualize and desire, it is necessary to act towards your goals. Set goals, create plans, and act with confidence, following the guidance of your intuition and your inner guide.

Co-creating with the Universe:

Arcturian Manifestation and Co-creation teaches us to co-create our reality in partnership with the universe, uniting our intention and action with the creative energy of the cosmos. Trust the flow of life, follow your intuition and act with confidence, knowing that the universe conspires in your favor to manifest your dreams.

Techniques for Manifestation:

- **Goal Setting:** Set clear and specific goals for your dreams, breaking them down into smaller steps and setting deadlines to achieve them.
- **Visualization Board:** Create a visualization board with images, phrases, and symbols that represent your dreams and goals. Look at your board daily, visualizing your dreams as if they were already reality.
- **Affirmations:** Use positive affirmations that express your desires and strengthen the belief in your ability to manifest your dreams.
- **Meditation:** Meditate with the intention of connecting with the energy of creation and visualizing your dreams manifesting.
- **Action:** Act towards your goals, taking concrete steps that bring you closer to realizing your dreams.

Arcturian Manifestation and Co-creation empowers you to create the life you desire, using the power of intention, visualization, gratitude, and action. By connecting with the creative energy of the universe and following the guidance of the

Arcturians, you will be manifesting your dreams with clarity, confidence, and joy, co-creating a reality of abundance, happiness, and fulfillment.

Chapter 45
Energy Exercises

Arcturian Energy Exercises offer a powerful tool to revitalize the energy body, harmonize emotions, and expand the connection with universal energy. The practice of these conscious movements promotes balance and well-being by activating the flow of vital energy that runs through the channels and centers of the subtle body, such as the chakras and meridians. This approach combines physical movement, intentional breathing, and visualization, allowing you to experience a state of integration between the physical, emotional, and spiritual body. By cultivating this energetic connection, you strengthen not only your vitality, but also your ability to align with the harmony and abundance of the universe.

The starting point for practice is to understand the dynamics of the energy body, which acts as an interconnected system. When energy flows freely, health and balance are maintained, but energy blocks can lead to emotional and physical discomfort. Simple exercises, such as Aura Breathing, help strengthen the protective layer of the energy body, creating a luminous field that keeps negative influences at bay. In addition, Chakra Activation allows for complete harmonization, promoting a sense of alignment and clarity in all dimensions of being.

Incorporating these practices into your routine does not require long sessions, but rather consistency and presence. An Energy Walk, performed in a natural environment, can be deeply restorative, while exercises such as Energy Stretching help release tension and energize the meridians. Energy Dance invites spontaneity and creative expression, unlocking patterns of stagnation and bringing a sense of lightness and joy. These moments of energetic care not only rejuvenate the body, but also expand perception and strengthen the connection with the cosmos.

With regular practice, Arcturian Energy Exercises become a way to explore inner vitality and the unlimited potential for balance and well-being. By integrating these movements into your daily life, you open yourself to a fuller life experience, rooted in harmony, flow, and deep connection with the universe and your own essence.

The Arcturians, with their deep understanding of energy anatomy, teach us that conscious movement is essential for health and well-being. Through energy exercises, we can activate the flow of vital energy (prana) in our body, harmonize the chakras, strengthen the aura, and expand our consciousness. Arcturian Energy Exercises combine physical movements, conscious breathing, and visualization, creating a powerful synergy that promotes balance, vitality, and connection with universal energy.

Understanding the Energy Body:

The energy body is a complex network of channels and energy centers that interpenetrates the physical body, influencing our health, our emotions, and our consciousness. The chakras, meridians, and aura are important components of the energy body, and the practice of energy exercises helps to maintain the free and harmonious flow of energy, promoting integral well-being.

Exercises to Strengthen the Energy Field:
- **Aura Breathing:** Stand with your feet shoulder-width apart, breathe deeply, and visualize your aura expanding with each inhale, enveloping your entire body in a sphere of light. Exhale slowly, feeling your aura contract and strengthen. Repeat the exercise for a few minutes, visualizing your aura vibrant and luminous.
- **Chakra Activation:** Sit or lie down comfortably, breathe deeply, and focus your attention on each chakra, starting with the root chakra and going up to the crown chakra. Visualize each chakra as a wheel of energy spinning

clockwise, vibrating with its corresponding color. Feel the energy flowing freely through each chakra, harmonizing and balancing your energy body.
- **Energy Stretching:** Stand with your feet shoulder-width apart, raise your arms overhead, and stretch your entire body as if you were trying to reach the sky. Breathe deeply, visualizing energy flowing from the earth to the sky through your body, stretching and energizing your meridians. Repeat the exercise to the sides, forward and backward, feeling the flexibility and vitality of your energy body.
- **Energy Walk:** Walk in a natural environment, such as a park or forest, focusing on your breathing and visualizing the energy of the earth rising through your feet and filling your entire body. Feel the connection with nature and the vitality that emanates from the earth.
- **Energy Dance:** Put on music that inspires you and dance freely, allowing your body to move with the music, expressing your energy and creativity. Visualize energy flowing through you, harmonizing your chakras and expanding your aura.

Benefits of Energy Exercises:
- **Increased Vitality:** Energy exercises increase vitality, energy, and physical disposition.
- **Energy Balance:** Harmonize the chakras, balance the subtle bodies, and promote the free flow of vital energy.
- **Strengthening the Aura:** Strengthen the aura, creating a protective shield against negative energies and dense influences.
- **Expansion of Consciousness:** Expand consciousness, increasing perception, intuition, and connection with the universe.
- **Relaxation and Well-being:** Promote relaxation, reduce stress, and increase feelings of well-being.

Incorporate Arcturian Energy Exercises into your daily routine, spending a few minutes a day to strengthen your energy body, increase your vitality, and deepen your connection to universal energy. With regular practice, you will feel the benefits in your physical, emotional, and spiritual health, treading a path of balance, harmony, and well-being.

Chapter 46
Mantras and Affirmations

The Arcturian Mantras and Affirmations reveal the profound transformative power of sound and words, essential tools for aligning thoughts and emotions with the highest frequencies of the universe. The practice of mantras not only harmonizes the energy field but also strengthens the spiritual connection, allowing you to access expanded states of consciousness and align with the loving and healing energy of the Arcturians. Affirmations, when used consistently and intentionally, reprogram the subconscious mind, promoting positive beliefs that drive the manifestation of your desires and the construction of a fuller reality aligned with the soul's purpose.

Mantras function as vibrational codes, each sound generating a specific resonance that reverberates in the energy body, harmonizing chakras and clearing blockages. When chanted with mindfulness, Arcturian mantras channel high energies of healing, love, and wisdom directly into your energy field, creating synergy between you and the cosmic forces. Chanting a mantra, like the powerful "OM," is like activating a key that opens the doors to balance and inner serenity, allowing you to connect with the universal flow of energy and receive the benefits of this attunement.

Affirmations complement this process by acting directly on mental patterns. By repeating phrases like "I manifest my dreams with ease and joy," you not only redefine your inner beliefs but also direct your energy to create the reality you desire. This practice is even more potent when combined with creative visualizations and genuine emotions, creating a vibration that magnetizes what is in tune with your intentions. By incorporating these tools into your routine, you not only strengthen your mind and spirit but also build a vibrational state aligned with abundance, healing, and fulfillment.

Uniting mantras and affirmations in your journey is like creating an energy field where each word chanted or affirmed resonates with purpose and strength. With regular practice and dedication, these techniques become powerful catalysts for personal transformation, helping you harmonize your being, raise your vibration, and manifest a life filled with love, light, and abundance.

The Arcturians, masters of the art of vibrational healing, understand the power of sound and words as instruments of healing and transformation. Mantras, sacred words or phrases, emit vibrations that raise consciousness, harmonize the chakras, and connect the human being with higher energies. Affirmations, positive and empowering phrases, reprogram the subconscious mind, replacing limiting beliefs with beliefs that drive growth and fulfillment. Arcturian Mantras and Affirmations combine the ancestral wisdom of sound with the loving and healing energy of the Arcturians, creating a powerful synergy that promotes healing, transformation, and conscious manifestation.

The Power of Mantras:

Mantras are words or phrases with vibrational power that, when chanted with intention and concentration, generate resonance with higher energies, promoting healing, harmonization, and expansion of consciousness. Arcturian mantras connect with the vibration of Arcturus, channeling energies of healing, love, and wisdom to your being.

Some Arcturian Mantras:
- **OM:** The universal mantra that represents the primordial vibration of the universe, connecting you with the divine source.
- **AUM:** A powerful mantra that activates the chakras and raises the vibration.
- **OM MANI PADME HUM:** The mantra of compassion, which purifies the heart and promotes emotional healing.

- **RA MA DA SA SA SAY SO HUNG:** A healing mantra that invokes vital energy and promotes physical well-being.
- **OM NAMAHA SHIVAYA:** A mantra that invokes the energy of Shiva, the god of transformation, promoting the release of limiting patterns.

Chanting the Mantras:
- **Intention:** Set the intention for the mantra practice, be it healing, protection, connection with the Arcturians, or manifestation.
- **Concentration:** Focus on the vibration of the mantra, feeling the vibrations resonating in your body and mind.
- **Repetition:** Repeat the mantra aloud or mentally, maintaining rhythm and concentration.
- **Visualization:** Visualize the energy of the mantra flowing through you, harmonizing your chakras and raising your vibration.

The Power of Affirmations:

Affirmations are positive and empowering phrases that, when repeated with conviction, reprogram the subconscious mind, replacing limiting beliefs with beliefs that drive growth and fulfillment. Arcturian affirmations connect with the energy of Arcturus, strengthening self-confidence, positivity, and the ability to manifest your dreams.

Examples of Arcturian Affirmations:
- "I am a being of light, connected with the energy of Arcturus."
- "I am healed and harmonized on all levels of my being."
- "I manifest my dreams with ease and joy."
- "I am prosperous and abundant in all areas of my life."
- "I live in peace, love and harmony with the universe."

Using Affirmations:
- **Repetition:** Repeat the affirmations daily, aloud or mentally, with conviction and emotion.

- **Visualization:** Visualize yourself living the reality you want to create, feeling the emotions as if your dreams were already reality.
- **Writing:** Write your affirmations in a journal, repeating them several times and visualizing them manifesting in your life.

Arcturian Mantras and Affirmations are powerful tools for co-creating your reality, transforming your thoughts, emotions, and beliefs. By using these tools with intention and consistency, you will be raising your vibration, manifesting your dreams and walking a path of light, love and abundance.

Chapter 47
Creative Visualizations

Arcturian Creative Visualizations unlock the immense power of the human mind to shape reality, transforming thoughts and intentions into concrete experiences. The practice uses imagination as a bridge between the inner world and external manifestations, allowing you to co-create your life with clarity and purpose. This technique is based on the principle that what we visualize with emotion and clear intention sends an energetic signal to the universe, aligning circumstances, people, and opportunities to bring to life what we desire. Through the energy and wisdom of the Arcturians, this practice becomes even more powerful, connecting you to the highest frequencies of healing and manifestation.

The basis of creative visualization lies in the ability to create vivid and detailed mental images, charged with positive emotions. When you imagine a goal as if it were already reality, your subconscious mind is reprogrammed to align thoughts, behaviors, and decisions with this new reality. This process is amplified by integrating all the senses during visualization—seeing, hearing, feeling, smelling, and even tasting what you want to manifest. The richer and more emotionally engaging the visualization, the greater the impact on the energy field and your connection to the universe.

In addition to promoting the manifestation of desires, creative visualization is a powerful tool for healing. On the physical level, you can visualize vital energy flowing through your body, regenerating cells and restoring balance. On the emotional plane, images of light and harmony help release traumas and fill the heart with love and serenity. Mentally, visualization can dispel limiting beliefs and cultivate a state of peace and clarity. These practices are enhanced by Arcturian energy, which guides and amplifies the effects of your intention.

To make the most of creative visualizations, create a space of tranquility and begin with deep relaxation. Set a clear intention for each practice and use positive affirmations to reinforce confidence in the manifestation of your desire. Regular repetition of visualization strengthens the mental image, creates a stronger energetic connection with the universe, and accelerates the co-creation process. With dedication and practice, you will develop the ability to transform dreams into reality, harnessing the power of imagination to heal, transform and co-create a life of fulfillment and accomplishment.

The Arcturians, with their advanced understanding of the human mind and universal laws, recognize creative visualization as a powerful tool for co-creating reality. The human mind is a portal to creation, a fertile field where the seeds of our thoughts and emotions germinate and manifest in our lives. Through creative visualization, you direct the power of your mind to create vivid images, charged with emotion and intention, that connect with the energy of the universe and materialize your dreams.

Understanding the Power of the Mind:

The human mind is a powerful instrument, capable of creating wonderful realities or trapping us in cycles of limitation and suffering. Arcturian Creative Visualization invites us to take control of our minds, using them as a tool for healing, transformation, and manifestation. By directing your thoughts, emotions, and mental images towards creating the reality you desire, you become a conscious co-creator of your destiny.

Creative Visualization in Arcturian Healing:

The Arcturians use creative visualization in their healing techniques, assisting in:

- **Physical Healing:** Visualize your body healing, your organs functioning in perfect harmony and vital energy flowing freely through each cell.

- **Emotional Healing:** Visualize your emotions balancing, releasing past traumas and hurts and filling your heart with love, peace and joy.
- **Mental Healing:** Visualize your mind calm and serene, free from negative thoughts and limiting beliefs, filled with clarity, focus and creativity.
- **Manifestation:** Visualize your dreams manifesting, feeling the emotions and sensations as if they were already reality.

Creative Visualization Techniques:
- **Relaxation:** Start with deep relaxation, calming the mind and body to facilitate concentration and visualization.
- **Intention:** Define the intention for your visualization, be it healing, transformation or manifestation.
- **Image Creation:** Create a vivid and detailed mental image of what you want to manifest, using all your senses: sight, hearing, touch, smell and taste.
- **Emotion:** Feel the emotions as if your wish were already reality, intensifying the energy of your visualization.
- **Affirmations:** Use positive affirmations that reinforce your visualization and strengthen the belief in the realization of your dreams.
- **Repetition:** Practice visualization regularly, repeating it several times a day to strengthen the mental image and connection with the energy of the universe.

Guided Visualizations by the Arcturians:

The Arcturians can guide you in creative visualizations, leading you through images, symbols and messages that amplify the power of your mind and facilitate the manifestation of your dreams. Connect with the Arcturians through meditation, invoke their presence and ask them to assist you in your visualizations.

Developing Imagination:

Imagination is the key to creative visualization. Cultivate your imagination through reading, art, music and contact with nature. The more you stimulate your imagination, the more powerful your ability to visualize and manifest your dreams will be.

Arcturian Creative Visualizations invite you to co-create your reality, using the power of your mind and the energy of the universe. By mastering visualization techniques, you will be transforming your dreams into reality, healing your being and manifesting a life of fullness, joy and fulfillment.

Chapter 48
Arcturian Rituals

Arcturian Rituals offer a transformative opportunity to access the sacred, align with high energies, and co-create positive changes in your life. These rituals channel the energy of the Arcturians, combining intention, symbolic elements, and meditative practices to create a bridge between the material and spiritual worlds. Through these conscious acts, you can promote healing, protection, and manifestation, while strengthening your connection to the universe and the ancestral wisdom of Arcturus.

One of the pillars of this practice is the Arcturian altar, which serves as a sacred space and an energy portal. Creating this altar is an act of intention: each element chosen—crystals, symbols, candles, colors or personal objects—reflects your connection to the Arcturians and your spiritual purposes. By activating this space with the energy of your daily practice, you establish an anchor point for your spiritual journey, reinforcing the presence of Arcturian energies in your life.

Rituals can be adapted to your needs and desires, from healing emotional wounds to protection from negative influences. A healing ritual, for example, may involve crystals carefully positioned on your chakras, accompanied by a visualization of light flowing through the body, transmuting dense energies and restoring balance. Protection rituals, on the other hand, create energy barriers, using tools such as white light or protective crystals, while you invoke the presence of the Arcturians to strengthen your aura. To manifest your dreams, the integration of creative visualizations and elements such as the energy of the New Moon or a visualization board intensifies the impact of your intentions.

The magic of Arcturian Rituals lies in repetition, focus and faith in the transformative power of practice. Incorporating them into your routine not only raises your vibration, but also connects you to a continuous flow of universal energy, promoting balance, abundance and harmony. Whether to heal, protect or manifest, rituals become a powerful expression of your role as a conscious co-creator of your reality, allowing you to live in a more aligned, meaningful and fulfilling way.

The Arcturians, with their deep connection to spirituality and universal energy, understand the power of rituals as tools for connecting with the Divine, for healing and transformation. Rituals are symbolic acts that create a sacred space, where intention, energy and consciousness unite to manifest your desires and co-create your reality. Arcturian Rituals combine the ancestral wisdom of rituals with the loving and healing energy of the Arcturians, creating a powerful synergy that amplifies the connection with the universe, raises the vibration and opens the way for the realization of your dreams.

Creating your Arcturian Altar:

The altar is a sacred space, a portal for connection with the Arcturians and with universal energy. To create your Arcturian altar, choose a quiet and special place in your home where you can connect with the energy of the Arcturians and perform your rituals. Decorate your altar with elements that represent Arcturus and Arcturian healing, such as:

- **Crystals:** Use crystals that amplify Arcturian energy, such as clear quartz, amethyst, selenite and Arcturian crystal (if you have access to it).
- **Images:** Use images that represent the Arcturians, such as paintings, drawings or photos of channeling.
- **Symbols:** Use Arcturian symbols, such as the Arcturus Star, the Sacred Triangle and the Golden Spiral.
- **Colors:** Use the colors that represent Arcturus, such as blue, violet and white.
- **Candles:** Use candles to illuminate your altar and represent Arcturian light and energy.

- **Incense:** Use incense with aromas that bring you peace, harmony and connection with the spiritual.
- **Flowers:** Use flowers to bring beauty and vitality to your altar.
- **Personal Objects:** Add personal objects that have meaning to you and that represent your dreams and aspirations.

Healing Rituals:

Arcturian healing rituals use the energy of the Arcturians, crystals, symbols and your intention to promote physical, emotional and spiritual healing. You can create your own healing rituals, adapting them to your needs and intuitions. Some examples of healing rituals:

- **Crystal Healing Ritual:** Place crystals on the chakras or areas of the body that need healing, invoke the energy of the Arcturians and visualize the healing energy flowing through the crystals and harmonizing your being.
- **Violet Flame Healing Ritual:** Invoke the Violet Flame, an energy of transmutation and healing, and visualize it surrounding your body, transmuting dense energies and promoting healing on all levels.
- **Angel Healing Ritual:** Invoke the presence of angels and ask them to assist you in physical, emotional and spiritual healing. Visualize the angels surrounding you with their wings of light, bringing healing and harmonization.

Protection Rituals:

Arcturian protection rituals create an energy shield around you, protecting you from negative energies, dense influences and psychic attacks. You can create your own protection rituals using the energy of the Arcturians, crystals and your intention. Some examples of protection rituals:

- **White Light Protection Ritual:** Visualize yourself surrounded by a sphere of white light, asking the Arcturians to protect you from any negative energy.

- **Crystal Protection Ritual:** Use protective crystals, such as black tourmaline, obsidian and smoky quartz, to create an energy shield around you.
- **Symbol Protection Ritual:** Draw or visualize protective symbols, such as the pentagram, the ankh cross and the Star of David, to strengthen your aura and protect yourself from negative energies.

Manifestation Rituals:

Arcturian manifestation rituals use the energy of the Arcturians, the Law of Attraction and the power of your intention to manifest your dreams and desires. You can create your own manifestation rituals, adapting them to your goals and intuitions. Some examples of manifestation rituals:

- **Vision Board Manifestation Ritual:** Create a vision board with images, phrases and symbols that represent your dreams and desires. Perform a ritual at your Arcturian altar, visualizing your dreams manifesting and feeling the emotion of fulfillment.
- **Crystal Manifestation Ritual:** Use crystals that amplify the energy of manifestation, such as citrine, pyrite and green quartz, to energize your desires and attract prosperity.
- **New Moon Manifestation Ritual:** The New Moon is an auspicious time to start new projects and manifest your dreams. Perform a ritual on the New Moon, writing your wishes on a piece of paper and burning it in a candle, while visualizing your dreams coming true.

Rituals are powerful tools for connecting with the energy of the universe, manifesting your desires and co-creating your reality. Incorporate Arcturian rituals into your life, creating a sacred space in your home, performing healing, protection and manifestation rituals, and experiencing the magic of connecting with the Arcturians in your daily life.

Chapter 49
Arcturian Cards

The wisdom of the Arcturian Cards is revealed as a powerful instrument of spiritual connection, providing clarity and guidance in moments of personal transformation. This set of cards channels the energy of Arcturus and the Arcturian masters, offering profound and healing messages that assist in aligning with your highest essence. Each card, carefully illustrated and imbued with symbolic meaning, acts as a bridge between you and the universal teachings, helping to illuminate paths, resolve doubts, and bring harmony to the areas of your life that need attention. The process involves not only interpretation but also a deep encounter with your intuition, guided by the energy of the Arcturians.

By interacting with these cards, you open yourself to a transcendental experience of learning and healing. Preparation for this moment is essential and involves practices such as meditation and visualization, which strengthen the attunement with the Arcturian frequency. The act of shuffling and selecting the cards goes beyond a mechanical gesture; it is a ritual of intention and connection, where each movement reflects the openness to receive the messages from the masters. By observing the symbols, keywords, and messages of the cards, Arcturian wisdom manifests, allowing you to understand the challenges and possibilities ahead, while expanding your intuitive perception.

Regular use of the Arcturian Cards offers a unique opportunity for personal and spiritual growth. Through them, you can explore themes ranging from emotional and spiritual healing to discovering your life purpose and overcoming inner barriers. Each interaction is an invitation to deepen self-knowledge and strengthen trust in your own intuition while building a meaningful connection with the Arcturians. These cards not only serve as an oracle but as an instrument to activate your innate ability to access universal wisdom, promoting transformation, balance, and evolution in your spiritual journey.

What are the Arcturian Cards?

The Arcturian Cards are a set of cards illustrated with symbols, images, and channeled messages from the Arcturians, created to assist in connecting with the wisdom and healing energy of Arcturus. Each card has a specific meaning that connects with different aspects of life, such as love, relationships, work, spirituality, healing, and soul purpose. By using the Arcturian Cards, you open a communication channel with the Arcturians, receiving messages, insights, and guidance for your challenges, doubts, and decisions.

Connecting with the Energy of the Cards:

Before using the Arcturian Cards, it is important to connect with the energy of Arcturus and the wisdom of the Arcturians. You can do this through meditation, visualization, or invocation. Hold the cards in your hands, feel their subtle energy, and ask the Arcturians to guide you in interpreting the messages.

Using the Arcturian Cards:

- **Formulate a Question:** Before shuffling the cards, formulate a clear and specific question about the area of your life where you want to receive guidance.
- **Shuffle the Cards:** Shuffle the cards with attention and intention, focusing on your question and asking the Arcturians to guide you in choosing the right card.
- **Choose a Card:** Choose a card from the deck, trusting your intuition and the guidance of the Arcturians.
- **Interpretation:** Observe the image, symbols, and keywords of the card. Reflect on the meaning of the card in relation to your question, seeking to understand the message that the Arcturians bring you.

- **Intuition:** Trust your intuition to interpret the message of the card, allowing your inner wisdom to guide you in understanding its meanings.

Types of Arcturian Cards:

There are different types of Arcturian Cards, each with its specific focus and purpose. Some examples:

- **Healing Cards:** Focused on issues of physical, emotional, and spiritual healing.
- **Relationship Cards:** Bring messages and insights about romantic, family, and social relationships.
- **Soul Purpose Cards:** Assist in discovering and fulfilling your soul purpose.
- **Ascension Cards:** Offer guidance and support in the spiritual ascension process.

Benefits of Arcturian Cards:

- **Self-knowledge:** Arcturian Cards assist in self-knowledge, bringing clarity about your patterns, beliefs, and challenges.
- **Guidance:** They offer guidance and direction for your challenges, doubts, and decisions.
- **Healing:** They bring messages of healing and harmonization to different areas of your life.
- **Connection with the Arcturians:** Strengthen your connection with the Arcturians, allowing you to receive their wisdom and guidance.
- **Intuition:** Stimulate the development of intuition and connection with your inner wisdom.

Creating your own Oracle:

You can also create your own Arcturian oracle using images, symbols, and messages that resonate with you and the energy of Arcturus. Use your creativity and intuition to create a personalized oracle that will assist you in your journey of self-knowledge and healing.

Conclusion:

The Arcturian Cards are a portal to the wisdom and healing energy of Arcturus, a guide on your journey of self-discovery, healing, and transformation. By using the cards with respect, intention, and intuition, you will be opening a communication channel with the Arcturians, receiving messages, insights, and guidance to walk your path of light.

Chapter 50
Ethics in Healing

The practice of healing is a sacred act that requires responsibility, integrity, and deep respect for the dignity and free will of each being. By positioning ourselves as channels of healing, we assume the commitment to act with pure intention and impeccable ethics, recognizing that our role is not to control or impose results, but to offer compassionate and loving support in each individual's process. Healing energy, especially in the Arcturian context, flows in harmony with universal wisdom, guided by principles that value collaboration, compassion, and recognition of human and spiritual limits.

One of the most important foundations in healing is respect for free will. Every human being has the right to choose their path, their experiences, and the rhythm of their own evolution. The role of the healer is to offer tools and support, without ever invading boundaries or imposing their beliefs and methods. This posture requires the healer to be attentive, free from ego, and focused on the genuine intention to serve the greater good. Through this approach, healing becomes not only an act of love but also a celebration of the autonomy and uniqueness of each journey.

Furthermore, ethics in healing includes a commitment to humility and compassion. The healer must recognize that they are only a channel, a facilitator of the energy that comes from higher dimensions and the inner strength of the person seeking healing. Humility allows the healer to remain open to continuous learning, while compassion creates a welcoming and safe environment where healing can occur at deeper levels. When these principles are integrated, the act of healing transcends techniques and methods, becoming an authentic expression of love and respect for the interconnection of all beings.

The Arcturians, with their advanced consciousness and deep compassion, teach us that healing is a sacred act, a loving service that aims at the well-being and evolution of all beings. Ethics in Arcturian Healing invites us to walk this path with responsibility, integrity, and respect, honoring the free will of each being and recognizing the limits of healing. It is an invitation to reflect on our own values, beliefs, and motivations, always seeking alignment with universal wisdom and the greater good.

Ethical Principles of Arcturian Healing:

- **Respect for Free Will:** Each being has the right to choose their own path, their own experiences, and their own healing process. The healer must respect the free will of each person, not imposing their beliefs, values, or methods, but offering healing as a path of support and assistance.
- **Pure Intention:** Healing must be performed with pure intention, aiming at the well-being of the person being healed and the greater good. The healer must be free from selfishness, vanity, and attachment to results, trusting in the wisdom of the universe and the healing process of each being.
- **Confidentiality:** Information shared during the healing process must be treated with confidentiality and respect. The healer must maintain secrecy about the personal and emotional issues of the person being healed, creating a safe and trusting space.
- **Humility:** The healer must recognize their limitations, understanding that they are only a channel for healing, and that true healing comes from inner strength and connection with the Divine. Humility allows the healer to be open to continuous learning, recognizing that healing is a process that involves collaboration between the healer, the person being healed, and the universe.

- **Compassion:** Compassion is the foundation of healing. The healer must approach the person being healed with love, empathy, and understanding, creating a space of welcome and support. Compassion allows the healer to connect with the other's pain, offering healing as a balm for the soul.
- **Responsibility:** The healer must take responsibility for their actions and the methods they use. It is important to seek knowledge, improve your techniques, and be aware of the limits of healing, referring the person to other professionals when necessary.

Limits of Healing:

It is important to recognize that healing is not a magical solution to all problems. There are limits to healing, and it is not always possible to achieve the expected results. The healer must be honest and transparent, explaining the limits of healing and not creating false expectations.

Healer's Responsibility:

The healer has the responsibility to:
- **Seek knowledge:** Improve their knowledge of healing techniques, energy anatomy, and the ethical principles of healing.
- **Take care of themselves:** Keep their own energy balanced and harmonized, taking care of their physical, emotional, and spiritual health.
- **Act with integrity:** Act with honesty, transparency, and respect in all their interactions.
- **Honor trust:** Maintain the confidentiality of information shared during the healing process.
- **Recognize their limits:** Recognize their limits and refer the person to other professionals when necessary.

Ethics in Arcturian Healing invites us to walk the path of healing with wisdom, responsibility, and compassion, honoring free will, dignity, and the evolutionary process of each being. By integrating ethical principles into your healing practice, you will be contributing to the creation of a more harmonious, loving, and conscious world, where healing manifests as a path of light and transformation.

Chapter 51
Healing and the Ascension Process

The practice of healing is a sacred act that requires responsibility, integrity, and deep respect for the dignity and free will of each being. By positioning ourselves as channels of healing, we assume the commitment to act with pure intention and impeccable ethics, recognizing that our role is not to control or impose results, but to offer compassionate and loving support in each individual's process. Healing energy, especially in the Arcturian context, flows in harmony with universal wisdom, guided by principles that value collaboration, compassion, and recognition of human and spiritual limits.

One of the most important foundations in healing is respect for free will. Every human being has the right to choose their path, their experiences, and the rhythm of their own evolution. The role of the healer is to offer tools and support, without ever invading boundaries or imposing their beliefs and methods. This posture requires the healer to be attentive, free from ego, and focused on the genuine intention to serve the greater good. Through this approach, healing becomes not only an act of love but also a celebration of the autonomy and uniqueness of each journey.

Furthermore, ethics in healing includes a commitment to humility and compassion. The healer must recognize that they are only a channel, a facilitator of the energy that comes from higher dimensions and from the inner strength of the person seeking healing. Humility allows the healer to remain open to continuous learning, while compassion creates a welcoming and safe environment where healing can occur at deeper levels. When these principles are integrated, the act of healing transcends techniques and methods, becoming an authentic expression of love and respect for the interconnection of all beings.

The Arcturians, with their panoramic vision of cosmic evolution, observe Earth and humanity with love and compassion, assisting us in this crucial moment of planetary ascension. Ascension is a process of raising vibration, expanding consciousness, and returning to unity with the divine source. It is a journey of profound transformation that affects all aspects of life, propelling humanity and the planet towards a new era of light, harmony, and consciousness.

The Interconnection between Healing and Ascension:

Healing and ascension are interconnected and complementary processes. Healing, on its various levels - physical, emotional, mental, and spiritual - prepares the ground for ascension, removing blockages, harmonizing energies, and raising vibration. Ascension, in turn, accelerates the healing process, paving the way for the manifestation of integral health and divine potential.

How Arcturian Healing Accelerates Ascension:

Arcturian healing, with its advanced technology and spiritual wisdom, acts as a catalyst for ascension, assisting in several aspects:

- **Raising Vibration:** Arcturian healing techniques raise individual and collective vibration, facilitating adaptation to the planet's new energy frequencies and paving the way for ascension.
- **Multidimensional Healing:** Arcturian healing works on all levels of being, releasing traumas, healing emotional wounds, expanding the mind, and strengthening the spiritual connection, preparing the individual for ascension.
- **DNA Activation:** Arcturian DNA activation awakens dormant light codes, expanding consciousness, accessing higher abilities, and accelerating the ascension process.
- **Connection with the Higher Self:** Arcturian healing strengthens the connection with the Higher Self, the

source of inner wisdom and guidance, assisting in making decisions aligned with the soul's purpose and the path of ascension.
- **Planetary Healing:** Arcturian planetary healing harmonizes telluric energies, purifies ecosystems, and promotes ecological balance, contributing to the ascension of the planet and all living beings.

Challenges and Opportunities of Ascension:

Planetary ascension is a challenging process that requires adaptation, transformation, and overcoming limiting patterns. However, it is also a unique opportunity for humanity to awaken to its true nature, manifest its divine potential, and co-create a new reality based on love, peace, and unity.

Some challenges of ascension:
- **Resistance to Change:** Attachment to old patterns, beliefs, and behaviors can generate resistance to change and hinder the ascension process.
- **Fears and Insecurities:** The intensification of planetary energy and the changes that accompany it can awaken fears and insecurities, generating anxiety and resistance.
- **Internal Conflicts:** Confrontation with shadows, traumas, and limiting patterns can generate internal conflicts and emotional challenges.

Some opportunities for ascension:
- **Expansion of Consciousness:** Ascension offers the opportunity to expand consciousness, access new dimensions of reality, and connect with universal wisdom.
- **Awakening of Divine Potential:** Ascension awakens the dormant divine potential in each human being, paving the way for the manifestation of gifts, talents, and higher abilities.
- **Co-creation of a New Reality:** Ascension invites us to be conscious co-creators of our reality, manifesting a future of peace, love, and harmony for humanity and the planet.

Conclusion:

Healing and the Arcturian Ascension Process invite us to walk the path of evolution with courage, trust, and love. By integrating Arcturian healing into your life, you will be preparing for ascension, raising your vibration, expanding your consciousness, and co-creating a new reality for yourself and the planet. Trust the wisdom of the Arcturians, surrender to the flow of life, and allow the loving energy of the universe to guide you on your ascension journey.

Chapter 52
Arcturian Community

The Arcturian Community represents a vibrant network of unity and spiritual growth, where souls who share similar values and aspirations connect to create an environment of learning, mutual support, and collective transformation. By participating in this community, you open yourself to experiences of exchange and expansion, driven by the loving and healing energy of the Arcturians. This network goes beyond simple sharing; it creates an energy field strengthened by the synergy of aligned intentions, providing a space for healing, individual growth, and the co-creation of a brighter reality.

Belonging to a spiritual community strengthens your journey of evolution by providing emotional, intellectual, and energetic support. In times of challenge, the exchange of experiences and perspectives can inspire solutions and renew confidence in the path. In addition, interaction with people who vibrate at the same frequency stimulates continuous learning, offering opportunities to share knowledge, explore new practices, and access valuable resources that enrich your spiritual understanding. In the Arcturian Community, each encounter is an opportunity to strengthen bonds of friendship and collaboration while walking towards common goals.

The collective energy generated by the community also amplifies the processes of healing and ascension. When individuals with similar purposes come together, a powerful magnetic field is created, capable of harmonizing energies and catalyzing transformations. In this space, dreams and intentions find fertile ground to flourish, while internal and external barriers dissolve. Actively participating in this network is more than joining a group; it is contributing to a larger movement of expansion of light and planetary consciousness, where each collaborative action strengthens the universal connection and raises the vibration of everyone involved.

The Arcturians, with their deep understanding of the interconnection between all beings, teach us that community is a fundamental pillar in the evolutionary journey. By joining with people who share our values, our dreams, and our search for healing and growth, we create a network of support, inspiration, and strength that propels us on our way. The Arcturian Community is a space of welcome, sharing, and learning, where you can connect with kindred souls, exchange experiences, receive support, and contribute to the expansion of light and consciousness on the planet.

Benefits of the Community:
- **Support and Inspiration:** The community offers support and inspiration in times of challenge, sharing experiences, offering different perspectives, and encouraging overcoming.
- **Learning and Growth:** The exchange of knowledge, experiences, and spiritual practices accelerates individual and collective learning and growth.
- **Strengthening the Connection:** The union of people who vibrate at the same frequency amplifies energy, strengthens the connection with the Arcturians, and facilitates the manifestation of dreams and goals.
- **Healing and Harmony:** The community creates an environment of healing and harmony, where energies are balanced, emotions are calmed, and consciousness expands.
- **Co-creation:** The union of souls seeking a better world facilitates the co-creation of a new reality, based on love, peace, and collaboration.

Connecting with the Arcturian Community:
- **Study Groups:** Look for Arcturian healing study groups in your city or online. Participate in meetings, lectures,

workshops, and courses to deepen your knowledge, share experiences, and connect with people who vibrate at the same frequency.
- **Online Resources:** Access websites, blogs, forums, and social networks that address Arcturian healing. Share your learning, ask questions, connect with other people, and participate in discussions on topics that interest you.
- **Events and Retreats:** Participate in events and retreats that promote Arcturian healing, meditation, spiritual development, and connection with nature. These events are opportunities to deepen your practice, receive healing, connect with people who share your interests, and strengthen bonds of friendship.
- **Create your own Community:** If you don't find a group that meets your needs, create your own Arcturian community. Gather friends, family, and people interested in Arcturian healing to share experiences, practice meditations, perform rituals, and co-create a space of light and love.

Contributing to the Community:
- **Share your Knowledge:** Share your knowledge, experiences, and learning with the community, contributing to the growth and expansion of all.
- **Offer Support:** Offer support to community members, sharing words of encouragement, offering help in times of difficulty, and celebrating each other's achievements and progress.
- **Participate Actively:** Actively participate in community activities, contributing ideas, suggestions, and actions that strengthen the group and promote unity.
- **Express Gratitude:** Express gratitude for the community, for the learning, for the support, and for the opportunity to connect with kindred souls.

The Arcturian Community is a network of light and love that connects you with people who vibrate at the same frequency, seeking healing, spiritual growth, and the co-creation of a better world. By connecting with the community, you will be expanding your horizons, strengthening your journey, and contributing to the expansion of light and consciousness on the planet. Together, we are stronger, wiser, and more capable of manifesting the reality we desire.

Chapter 53
Next Steps in Arcturian Healing

The ongoing journey of Arcturian healing is a call to explore new horizons of learning and evolution, integrating the teachings of the Arcturians into your life experience. Each step forward on this path represents an opportunity to deepen your self-knowledge, expand your consciousness, and act as a beacon of light in the world. Guided by the loving energy of the Arcturians, you are encouraged to open yourself to new practices, connections, and ways of sharing wisdom and healing with those around you, while strengthening your own spiritual transformation.

To move forward on this path, the first step is to invest in deepening your knowledge. There are a plethora of resources available that can enrich your understanding of Arcturian healing and your role as an agent of transformation. Books, courses, workshops, and lectures are valuable sources of learning, allowing you to explore advanced techniques, understand the fundamentals of sacred geometry and channeling, or learn about spiritual ascension in depth. In addition, the accompaniment of experienced mentors or spiritual guides can bring clarity and guidance, helping you to overcome blockages, refine your skills, and connect more deeply with the Arcturians and your Higher Self.

As your practice deepens, the expansion of consciousness becomes a priority. Dedicating yourself to daily rituals of meditation, visualization, and energetic connection strengthens your attunement to the Arcturian frequency and nourishes your ability to access higher dimensions of understanding. Regular contact with nature can complement this practice, providing balance, tranquility, and inspiration. At the same time, diving into your inner journey is essential to understanding your emotions, beliefs, and behavior patterns, helping to integrate important lessons and manifest the fullness of your potential.

As you strengthen yourself on this path, you are invited to share the light of healing with the world. This sharing can take many forms: offering healing to those seeking help, leading study and meditation groups, or participating in collective initiatives aimed at peace and planetary harmony. Each act of service is a way to multiply the light and strengthen the bonds of compassion and collaboration. Thus, the Arcturian journey becomes not only a path of personal evolution but also a significant contribution to the spiritual growth of humanity and the planet as a whole.

The journey of Arcturian healing is a continuous process of learning, growth, and transformation. By connecting with the energy of the Arcturians, you open the doors to a universe of possibilities, awakening to your true nature, healing your wounds, and manifesting your potential. The Next Steps in Arcturian Healing invite you to continue this journey, deepening your knowledge, expanding your consciousness, and sharing the light of healing with the world.

Deepening your Knowledge:
- **Books and Materials:** Explore the vast library of books, articles, and materials on Arcturian healing, spirituality, and personal development. Look for authors and channels that resonate with you, deepening your knowledge of the Arcturians, their healing techniques, and the principles of ascension.
- **Courses and Workshops:** Participate in courses and workshops on Arcturian healing, meditation, channeling, crystals, sacred geometry, and other topics that interest you. Learning from experienced masters and instructors accelerates your development and connects you with a community of people who share your quest for knowledge.

- **Mentors and Guides:** Seek guidance from mentors and spiritual guides who can assist you on your journey. An experienced mentor can offer support, clarity, and direction, helping you overcome challenges, integrate your learning, and manifest your potential.

Expanding your Consciousness:
- **Daily Practice:** Maintain a daily practice of meditation, energy healing, visualization, and connection with the Arcturians. Regular practice strengthens your connection with Arcturian energy, expands your consciousness, and accelerates your ascension process.
- **Experiences in Nature:** Connect with nature, seeking peace and harmony in natural environments. Nature is an inexhaustible source of healing and wisdom, which helps you connect with your essence and expand your consciousness.
- **Inner Journey:** Dedicate yourself to the inner journey, exploring your emotions, thoughts, and beliefs. Self-knowledge is fundamental for healing, growth, and ascension.
- **Loving Service:** Put your gifts and talents at the service of others, contributing to the healing of the planet and humanity. Loving service expands your consciousness, connects you with your soul's purpose, and accelerates your evolutionary journey.

Sharing the Light of Healing:
- **Share your Knowledge:** Share your knowledge and experiences with others, inspiring them to walk the path of healing and ascension.
- **Offer Healing:** If you feel called to be a healer, offer your services with love, compassion, and responsibility.
- **Create a Study Group:** Gather people interested in Arcturian healing to share knowledge, practice meditations, and perform group healing work.

- **Contribute to the Community:** Participate in projects and initiatives that promote healing, peace, and sustainability on the planet.

The journey of Arcturian healing is a unique and personal adventure. Trust your intuition, follow your heart, and create your own path, guided by the wisdom of the Arcturians and the light of your Higher Self. The Next Steps in Arcturian Healing invite you to continue this journey, deepening your knowledge, expanding your consciousness, and sharing the light of healing with the world. The future is yours to create!

Chapter 54
Arcturian Masters

Connecting with the Arcturian Masters opens doors to a journey of profound transformation, guided by beings of high consciousness and compassion. These masters act as beacons of light, radiating wisdom, unconditional love, and healing to those who seek to expand their spirituality and manifest their divine potential. By integrating with their energies, you access a vibrational field that stimulates your evolution, awakens inner wisdom, and strengthens your connection to the universe, allowing you to walk the path of ascension with confidence and purpose.

The Arcturian Masters are living examples of loving service to humanity, each contributing their unique energy to support our healing and spiritual awakening. They teach us that true evolution comes from the balance between knowledge and practice, between connection with the divine and compassion applied in the material world. By invoking and meditating with masters such as Juliano, Sananda, and Metatron, you begin to access higher levels of consciousness, where understanding expands beyond words and where healing manifests in a profound and transformative way.

This connection is not limited to meditation; it is an invitation to integrate the teachings of the Arcturian Masters into your daily life. The practice of unconditional love, the search for harmony with nature, and the study of spiritual principles, such as sacred geometry, become tools that help shape your journey. By recognizing your own multidimensionality and the power of love and forgiveness, you allow the light of the masters to guide your actions, inspire your choices, and strengthen your journey towards wholeness and alignment with divine purpose.

The Arcturian Masters are ascended beings who have transcended the limitations of the third dimension and are dedicated to loving service to humanity. They are like beacons of light that illuminate the path of ascension, sharing their wisdom and compassion to assist those who seek healing, self-knowledge, and connection with the Divine. Through connection with the Arcturian Masters, you can receive guidance, healing, and inspiration to walk your evolutionary path with more clarity, purpose, and love.

Juliano:

Juliano is an Arcturian ascended master known for his wisdom, compassion, and dedication to planetary healing. He is a loving guide who assists in connecting with the Gaia Consciousness, harmonizing telluric energies, and co-creating a sustainable future. Juliano teaches us to love and respect nature, to live in harmony with the planet, and to work together for the healing of the Earth. He reminds us that we are all interconnected and that our actions directly impact the health of the planet.

To connect with Juliano:
- Meditate: Visualize Juliano in his light form, feeling his loving and compassionate energy.
- Invoke his presence: Call on Juliano in your times of need, asking for his guidance and help.
- Connect with nature: Spend time in contact with nature, feeling the energy of Gaia and the presence of Juliano.

Sananda:

Sananda is the Christic consciousness that manifests through various avatars, including Jesus Christ. He represents unconditional love, compassion, and forgiveness, guiding humanity towards ascension and unity. Sananda teaches us to love ourselves and others, to forgive offenses, and to live in peace and harmony. He reminds us that we are all children of God, created in his image and likeness, and that love is the most powerful force in the universe.

To connect with Sananda:
- Meditate: Visualize Sananda in his light form, feeling his unconditional love and compassion.
- Invoke his presence: Call on Sananda in your times of need, asking for his healing and guidance.
- Practice unconditional love: Seek to love yourself and others unconditionally, expressing compassion, forgiveness, and kindness.

Metatron:

Metatron is an archangel and ascended master known for his cosmic wisdom and connection to sacred geometry. He assists in DNA activation, expansion of consciousness, and understanding the mysteries of the universe. Metatron teaches us to access our inner wisdom, connect with our divine essence, and manifest our full potential. He reminds us that we are multidimensional beings with unlimited capacities and potential.

To connect with Metatron:
- Meditate: Visualize Metatron in his light form, feeling his wisdom and power.
- Invoke his presence: Call on Metatron in your times of need, asking for his guidance and help.
- Study sacred geometry: Explore the patterns and symbols of sacred geometry, connecting with Metatron's cosmic wisdom.

Other Arcturian Masters:

In addition to Juliano, Sananda, and Metatron, there are many other Arcturian Masters who are dedicated to the healing and ascension of humanity. Explore their teachings, connect with their energies, and allow them to guide you on your evolutionary journey.

Integrating the Teachings of the Masters:
- Study: Study the teachings of the Arcturian Masters, deepening your knowledge of spirituality, healing, and ascension.

- Reflection: Reflect on the teachings of the masters, applying them in your daily life and seeking to integrate their wisdom into your actions and decisions.
- Practice: Practice the techniques and teachings of the masters, cultivating unconditional love, compassion, forgiveness, and wisdom in your daily life.

The Arcturian Masters are loving guides who accompany us on our evolutionary journey, offering their wisdom, healing, and inspiration. By connecting with the masters, you will be opening your heart to the light, love, and wisdom of the universe, walking the path of ascension with more clarity, purpose, and joy.

Chapter 55
The Future of Healing

The future of Arcturian healing reveals itself as a powerful convergence between science, spirituality, and the ancestral wisdom of the Arcturians, bringing a new paradigm for well-being and the evolution of humanity. In this future, healing is no longer just the elimination of symptoms but becomes a journey of energy harmonization and expansion of consciousness. Diseases are understood as manifestations of deeper imbalances and, through integrated approaches, body, mind, and spirit find alignment, promoting not only health but also the ascension of being.

Technology plays a revolutionary role in this context, acting as a catalyst for healing at deeper levels. Advanced tools, such as vibrational devices, personalized artificial intelligence, and therapeutic virtual reality, will transform diagnostic and treatment processes, making them more effective and accessible. Distance healing, facilitated by cutting-edge technologies, will transcend geographical barriers, ensuring that everyone has access to the necessary therapies. These technological innovations will always be aligned with spiritual principles, respecting the sacredness of the healing process and integrating it with the connection to the divine.

Furthermore, spirituality becomes the foundation for integral health, promoting practices that encompass self-knowledge, intuition, and connection with higher dimensions. Healing communities will emerge as spaces for the exchange of knowledge and experiences, fostering an environment of learning and collaboration. More conscious educational systems will teach about energy, self-healing, and spiritual practices, preparing future generations for a deeper understanding of well-being. This future will not just be about healing what is in imbalance, but also about cultivating a life of harmony, where healing is integrated as part of daily life and collective evolution.

The future of Arcturian healing will be, above all, a call for humanity to co-create a more conscious and enlightened world, where science and spirituality walk side by side. Each individual, by opening themselves to this vision, actively participates in the construction of a reality in which healing is not only individual, but also planetary, raising the frequency of the Earth and promoting peace and global sustainability.

The Arcturians, with their advanced technology and deep connection to the Divine Source, offer us a glimpse into the future of healing, a future where science and spirituality unite to create a new era of well-being for humanity. They show us that healing transcends the limits of the physical body, encompassing all levels of being - emotional, mental, and spiritual. In the future of healing, disease is understood as an energy imbalance, and healing becomes a process of harmonization, alignment, and raising vibration.

Technology at the Service of Healing:

In the future of healing, technology becomes a powerful ally in promoting well-being and ascension. Imagine:

- **Healing Devices:** Devices that use sound, light and vibrational frequencies to harmonize the chakras, balance the subtle bodies and promote healing at deep levels.
- **Artificial Intelligence in Healing:** Artificial intelligence systems that assist in the diagnosis and treatment of diseases, personalizing therapies and optimizing results.
- **Virtual Reality in Healing:** Immersive virtual reality experiences that promote emotional healing, trauma release, and the development of consciousness.
- **Distance Healing:** Technologies that allow healing at a distance, breaking the barriers of space and time, making healing accessible to everyone, regardless of location.

Spirituality as the Basis of Healing:

In the future of healing, spirituality becomes the basis for understanding health and well-being. Connection with the Divine, the development of intuition and the search for self-knowledge become pillars of integral healing. Imagine:

- **Spiritual Healing:** Techniques and practices that connect with divine energy, promoting the healing of the soul, the release of karmas and the awakening of consciousness.
- **Healing Communities:** Communities that come together to share knowledge, practice healing and co-create a more harmonious future.
- **Education for Healing:** Educational systems that teach about energy healing, self-healing and the importance of spiritual connection for health and well-being.

Healing as a Path of Evolution:

In the future of healing, healing becomes a path of evolution of consciousness, a process that transcends the simple elimination of symptoms and becomes a journey of self-discovery, transformation and ascension. Imagine:

- **Healing as a Lifestyle:** Healing becomes a lifestyle, where people dedicate themselves to self-knowledge, conscious eating, the practice of energy exercises and connection with nature.
- **Healing and Planetary Ascension:** Healing becomes an instrument for planetary ascension, harmonizing the energies of the Earth, raising collective consciousness and co-creating a future of peace and sustainability.
- **Conscious Humanity:** A humanity conscious of its interconnection with the universe, which uses healing as a tool for individual and collective evolution, co-creating a future of light, love and harmony.

The future of healing is in our hands. By integrating technology, spirituality and ancestral wisdom, we can co-create a future where healing becomes a path of light for the evolution of consciousness and the construction of a more harmonious and enlightened world. Trust the vision of the Arcturians, follow your intuition and contribute to the creation of a future where healing is accessible to all and propels us towards ascension.

Epilogue

Upon reaching the end of this journey, you are no longer the same. Something inside you has changed—a subtle but powerful transformation has occurred, an expansion of what you understand to be possible. The tools and practices presented here went far beyond what conventional reading could provide. This book, in its essence, was a bridge to awakening your own infinite potential.

The path you have walked on these pages does not end here. In fact, it unfolds in directions that only you can explore. Each technique, each symbol, each insight planted seeds of transformation that will continue to germinate. Just as the Arcturians teach, healing is not a destination, but a continuous journey of ascension and reconnection with the divine within you.

Now, you carry within you a new consciousness, a wisdom activated by Arcturian energies. Use it to create, to heal, to transform your reality. Allow the higher vibrations you have connected with to permeate all aspects of your life. No matter where you are, the connection with the Arcturians remains alive. They guide, inspire and celebrate every step of your progress.

Remember: the light you have awakened in yourself is not just for you. It is a gift to the world, a beacon that can inspire others to find their own healing and ascension. The universe is a vast field of interconnected energy, and your transformation resonates through it, touching lives and raising frequencies.

This book may have come to an end, but what it initiated in you is just the beginning. The journey continues, and you are both the traveler and the path. May Arcturian wisdom always guide you, and may you find in your own light the strength to walk towards fullness.

Be light. Be transformation. Be the healing the world awaits.

www.ingramcontent.com/pod-product-compliance
Lightning Source LLC
LaVergne TN
LVHW041924070526
838199LV00051BA/2718